LIFEP
DI

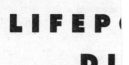

—

Peter Cox and Peggy Brusseau

THE LAST DIET BOOK
YOU'LL EVER READ . . .
OR NEED!

BLOOMSBURY

Publisher's Note
LifePoints and the LifePoints logo are protected by international copyright, trade mark and service mark legislation and may only be used with the express permission of the proprietor, The Alta Vista Corporation Ltd.

The information in this book was correct to the best of the Editor's and Publisher's belief at the time of going to press. While no responsibility can be accepted for errors and omissions, the Editor and Publisher would welcome corrections and suggestions for material to include in subsequent editions of this book.

This book may include words, brand names and other descriptions of products which are or are asserted to be proprietary names or trademarks. No judgement concerning the legal status of such words is made or implied thereby. Their inclusion does not imply that they have acquired for legal purposes a non-proprietary or general significance nor any other judgement concerning their legal status.

This edition first published in 1996 by
Bloomsbury Publishing plc
2 Soho Square
London, W1V 6HB

Copyright © by Peter Cox and Peggy Brusseau 1996

The moral right of the authors has been asserted

A copy of the CIP entry for this book is available from the British Library

ISBN 0 7475 2166 2

Typeset by Hewer Text Composition Services, Edinburgh
Printed and bound in Great Britain by
Cox & Wyman Ltd, Reading

AN IMPORTANT NOTE TO OUR READERS

All diets should begin with a medical check-up to make certain that no special health problems exist and to confirm that there are no medical reasons why you should not undertake a change of diet. Because the diagnosis and treatment of medical conditions is a responsibility shared between you and your medical advisors, neither the authors nor publisher of this book can accept responsibility for the individual consequences of dietary treatment based on the recommendations described herein.

The LifePoints system as described in this book has been created to be used by healthy adults only. It does not apply to pregnant or lactating women, or to children. Women who are pregnant or lactating should not consider any weight-reduction diet until they have returned to a non-pregnant, non-lactating condition. A reduction in protein intake is emphatically not recommended for a woman who is pregnant or lactating as the health of her child relies on both a higher-protein and higher-calorie intake during this time.

Also by Peter Cox and Peggy Brusseau:

LifePoints
The revolutionary guide to the goodness in
food – 'The diet revolution of the decade!' . . . Daily Mail

LifePoints Cookbook
A delicious collection of over 150 quick and easy recipes,
high in LifePoints and very low in RiskPoints.

LifePoints For Kids
Helps parents everywhere to choose the RIGHT food
for their children.

A Free Offer to our Readers

Peter Cox is the editor of *The Superliving Letter*, a unique
newsletter which covers the latest developments in food
and nutrition, health and healing, and personal growth. If
you would like to receive a free copy together with
subscription details, please send your name and address
with two first-class stamps to: The Superliving Letter,
PO Box 1612, London NW3 1TD

CONTENTS

TAKE THE LIFEPOINTS TEST DRIVE!

Most diet books are full of endless explanations, exhortations, complications and mitigations! If you're fed up with all that, you can prove to yourself right now just how revolutionary the new LifePoints system is . . . No need to read any further for the moment – just do it!

1   Turn to pages 167–238 and browse through the list of foods until you find one or two you'd like to eat during the day.

2   Jot down their LifePoints and RiskPoints numbers. LifePoints are a measure of the food's health-enhancing nutrients. RiskPoints are a measure of the food's harmful ingredients. So: you should aim to choose foods which have a *high* LifePoints number and a *low* RiskPoints number.

3   Continue to add further foods from the list, choosing as widely as possible from the first four groups. Gradually adjust your diet: your total RiskPoints per day should *not* exceed 100; your total LifePoints per day *must* be greater than 100.

Now you know how phenomenally easy the LifePoints system is! Can you imagine yourself using it to plan a really healthy diet? Of course! Why don't you experiment with it for a few minutes, perhaps checking up on some of your favourite foods, and then – when you're ready – turn to Part One to learn more about the world's simplest and most powerful food control system!

INTRODUCTION

Welcome to the world's simplest and most powerful food control system!

If you want to make friends with your food, and are fed up with feeling that each meal is a trial of will-power, then LifePoints can help.

If you're wrestling with a weighty waistline, and want to shed those surplus pounds safely and surely, then LifePoints can help.

And if you want your diet to provide you with an abundance of the vital nutrients which can safeguard your health and protect against many of today's most common afflictions – then Life-Points can help you do that too.

We created the original LifePoints system because we wanted to use it ourselves as a road map to healthy eating. We're delighted to report that, since the first LifePoints book was published, many people have been in touch to say how useful they find it as they navigate through their daily food choices. One of the most gratifying endorsements we've received came from Dr Neal Barnard, President of the Physicians Committee for Responsible Medicine, who wrote: 'LifePoints is an elegantly simple and extremely practical guide based on sound scientific principles. It will help you make nutritional choices that will revolutionize your health.'

But it also became clear that many people wanted us to go further, and show them how the LifePoints system can be used to achieve the trimming and slimming they're looking for. And no wonder – official statistics show that in the past decade alone the number of overweight Americans has increased by 31 per cent, and the number of chubby Brits by a (literally!) staggering 50 per cent.[1] If you want to see something really alarming, just look at the way these figures are predicted to rise in the next few years, as summarized on pages 9–10.

Why will the LifePoints Diet work for *you*? There are three major success factors which put the LifePoints system way ahead of all other diets:

First Success Factor: LifePoints is More Than a Diet

Let's face it – going on a diet is about as exciting as a trip to the dentist for root-canal work. But the hope of a trimmer, healthier you at the end of the painful dieting process usually motivates you to give it a try . . . for a time. The big problem, however, is that most conventional diets *don't* ultimately succeed. Maybe you can keep it up for a week or so; maybe for a month or more. But for six months, twelve months . . . a *lifetime*? Eventually your will-power cracks. End of diet . . . start of guilt! In a recent issue of the *British Medical Journal*, this is how researchers summed up the situation:

> It is well known that most treatments produce temporary weight loss. But it is equally well known that 90 per cent to 95 per cent of those who lose weight regain it within several years . . . We should stop offering ineffective treatments aimed at weight loss . . . Only by admitting that our treatments do not work – and showing that we mean it by refraining from offering them – can we begin to undo a century of recruiting fat people for failure.[2]

Today, there is new, and somewhat heartening, evidence to suggest that the '95 per cent failure' figure may be an over-estimate. That figure refers to people treated in hospital clinics. Recent research (see below) suggests that people who diet on their own – *not* under the supervision of a hospital or clinic – may actually be rather more successful with the failure rate only in the region of 75 per cent. Which is bad enough – but not *quite* so depressing!

> **You'll find lots of tips like this sprinkled throughout the book – while not part of the diet, the hints and person-to-person advice they contain may be very useful to you!**

Even so, the truth is that traditional diets usually fail, and they do so because they make unreasonable demands of you, and have no respect for your individuality or your personal food preferences. And when they *do* fail, they make it seem as if *you* are the one to blame. Not true! Feeling guilty about flunking a diet is about as logical as feeling responsible for tomorrow's weather. Diets fail *people* – not the other way around.

Because traditional diets have such a poor record of success, several consequences follow. One is the establishment of a burgeoning diet industry, which is now estimated to be worth a mind-boggling 33 *billion* dollars a year in the US.[3] Another is the understandable counter-reaction to this commercialism – a growing social trend termed the 'Size Acceptance Movement', which aims to oppose the unfair prejudice that larger folk often encounter. Research suggests that the overweight have to put up with discrimination in admission to universities, employment, promotion and access to housing, and earn, on average, $6,710 (£4,470) a year less than their slimmer colleagues.[4]

The LifePoints Diet cuts through all this. In the old-fashioned sense, it's not a 'diet' at all, because it doesn't make you eat small portions of unpleasant food for a brief time, before allowing you to 'relapse' to your previous ways of eating. Nor does it try to make you feel guilty about your size, weight, shape or condition. There's enough guilt around as it is! Instead, the LifePoints Diet is a very powerful tool which can help you to manage and control your lifetime's total food intake – your true 'diet'. And like all good and useful tools, it won't (and shouldn't) try to boss you around! With the LifePoints system, *you're* in control.

SECOND SUCCESS FACTOR: LIFEPOINTS IS HOLISTIC

As you'll see, the LifePoints Diet is not obsessed with calorie-counting. For decades, the entire diet industry has worshipped at the shrine of the sacrosanct calorie. Unfortunately, all they've managed to achieve in that time is a 95 per cent failure rate. Not a very good record, is it?

As you'll discover, there are many hidden dangers in strict calorie-counting, not the least of which is that it's virtually *impossible* to follow for any length of time – unless you have a brain like Einstein's and a will of iron. Most old-fashioned diets are only interested in crushing those troublesome calories – they aren't at all concerned with your overall nutrient intake. Just concentrating on one small aspect of your food intake is bound to lead to failure, and it routinely does.

By contrast, LifePoints takes a holistic view. The first priority of the LifePoints Diet is to ensure an optimum intake of essential nutrients. Indeed, we have come to the conclusion that the consistent pattern of over-eating displayed by some people may, in reality, be a desperate search for those essential nutrients that are lacking in much of today's foods.

To those people who are cruelly classified as 'diet failures', this holistic – and very positive – approach will come as a nice surprise! Most old-fashioned diets concentrate on telling you what you *can't* eat. Calorie-counting, in particular, makes you see virtually all food as a hazard. You know how it goes .... you're halfway through the day and you fancy a small snack. But can you squeeze another 175 calories into your day's allowance? Should you be naughty and 'pig-out' on something that's really off-limits? You feel your will-power quickly slipping away. OK, you tell yourself, just this once, but I'll be good tomorrow ... Argh! Calorie-counting makes you feel *bad* about food. That's appalling, because food is – and *should* be – one of life's main pleasures. LifePoints, on the other hand, makes you feel *good* about food. Together, we're going to raise our food expectations. Which leads us on to the third success factor ...

> **Never go to the supermarket hungry! People who shop on full stomachs can more easily resist those impulse buys of high-fat, low-nutrition food.**

THIRD SUCCESS FACTOR: LifePoints is Instinctive

We read a diet book recently which claimed that one of the biggest health threats faced by people today came from carrots. No, not the pesticide or other chemicals which might contaminate them – just plain, simple, common or garden carrots.

Well, everyone should have a right to express their views, no matter how goofy. But trying to make out that *carrots* are the root of all dietary evil is certifiable insanity!

This neatly illustrates the problem with most old-fashioned diets. In order to follow them, you're expected to ignore your own common sense and distrust your own instincts. No wonder most of them fail.

This is confirmed by research recently commissioned by the American Dietetic Association, who asked Gallup to conduct a survey into the nation's eating habits. Fully 46 per cent of the people questioned admitted that they found it difficult to eat healthily. The survey revealed that by far the biggest problem most people encountered was, simply, that healthy eating took too much time.[5] And the truth is, it usually does. If you're following a calorie-restricted diet, working out your daily food intake takes time – lots of it. Finding the right food in the shops takes time. Preparing it in a different way to the one you're used to takes even more time. And the main reason all this takes such a huge clump of your time is that it's not *instinctive*. You can understand why it's so much easier just to grab something familiar, and avoid the hassle of calorie-counters, shopping stupidity, and kitchen crises.

> **Shop to a plan! In the supermarket, first head for the fresh fruits and vegetables – if you fill your basket with healthy produce, you'll have less room for junk. Try to shorten your time in the centre aisles where the biscuits, sweets and crisps are.**

And now here's the good news! You'll notice something very different happens when you start the LifePoints Diet. It *sharpens your instincts* about food. Fundamentally, humans have a sound instinct about what constitutes nourishing food and what doesn't. After all, if we hadn't developed the ability to tell the difference between good food and bad, our species wouldn't have survived very long, would it? The problem is, our instincts can't always cope with the baffling and bewildering range of foods available nowadays, nor with the high-pressure ways in which many of these foods are sold.

We can explain this with a short example. Animals in their natural environment never die from over-eating – the greatest threat comes, of course, from starvation. Therefore, the best survival strategy is to eat whenever you've got the opportunity, because you never know where your next meal's coming from. That's why many of us *still* have the instinct to eat whenever we get the chance – even though our logical minds tell us that there is no conceivable likelihood of starving to death. The truth is that an instinct, which has served us well for at least 40,000 years, has

– within the last 100 years – become a major liability to us.

One of the most enjoyable aspects of the LifePoints Diet is that it will help you to *rediscover* your natural instincts about wholesome food and healthy eating. It'll encourage you to get in touch with your inborn discrimination, which helps us all – if we let it – distinguish excellence in nutritious food. It's an instinct that, once rediscovered, will stay with you for the rest of your life.

These three crucial factors make the LifePoints Diet unique. Now, you are barely seconds away from the start of your journey of discovery . . . We wish you every possible success, and hope you have as much fun on the way as we had blazing the trail. We promise you will never see food the same way again!

Peter Cox and Peggy Brusseau

PART ONE: LIFEPOINTS IS FOR LIFE!

If you ever happen to meet a diet book author, here's a very embarrassing question to ask: If diet books *really* worked, why are people fatter today than ever before?

The evidence for this is all around us. Two examples: when New York's Yankee Stadium was built in 1922 the width of the seats was set to a very generous 19 inches. Fifty years later, the American bottom had broadened so much that each seat had to be widened by 3 full inches. In Britain, an official report into the ability of firemen to do their job revealed that half of them were overweight, and 15 per cent so seriously obese that they couldn't perform their duties – such as climbing a ladder – without suffering from considerable physical stress. Throughout the Western world, in fact, the trend is clear: the future is fleshy.

The really disturbing information, though, comes from the rather dry national statistics which are released from time to time. Figure One shows the picture for British women. In the year 1980, one in three women (32 per cent) were officially classified as being overweight.[6] Since then, that figure has grown by about 1 per cent every year, so that 11 years later, 41 per cent of women fell into the overweight category. If the present trend continues – and there's no sign that it won't – the year AD 2002 will be something of a milestone. At that point, fully half of all British women – one in two – will be fatties. Perhaps we should have a national celebration: '2002, The Year of the Blob'. After that, of course, lean people will be in the minority, and will no doubt be discriminated against in the same way that overweight people have been in the past. And if you're wondering what the picture is for men, well, it's even worse. By 2002, fully 65 per cent of all males (two out of every three) will be chubbies. At least the women will have some company . . .

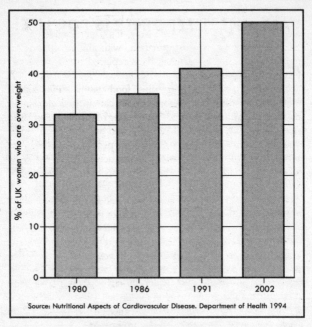

Source: Nutritional Aspects of Cardiovascular Disease. Department of Health 1994

Figure One: Heavy times ahead

> **When you get the sudden urge to binge, train yourself to wait 10 minutes before snacking – most food cravings disappear within that time.**

OF MICE AND GENES

While we're on the subject, let's make one thing very clear. Many people – sometimes doctors and scientists – refer to fatness as a genetic problem. This isn't surprising, because hardly a week goes by without news of some great medical breakthrough where researchers have discovered the gene for diabetes, alcoholism, bad breath or divorce. The impression often created is that humans are mere computers whose programming code – in this case, the genetic code – controls every aspect of our lives. This in turn makes us feel hopeless . . . after all, if you're 'born to be fat' there's nothing you can do about it, is there? In a way, it's a similar idea to the medieval concept of predestination, with the exception that today's white-coated scientists have replaced the deity as our source of salvation.

Like most statements regarding food, fatness and dieting, there's *some* truth in it. Some people can indeed eat almost anything and get away with it. At a meeting of the American Heart Association, Dr Francine K. Welty recited one such case. While doing a cholesterol-screening study on people with a high-fat, high-cholesterol diet, Dr Welty came across an 82-year-old father, five sons, and one daughter who regularly consumed 3,500 calories every day – almost half of them in the form of fat, and half of those in the form of saturated fat. Breakfast would consist of bacon and eggs, buttered toast or pancakes, cereal with whole milk, and coffee with cream. Heaven knows what they ate during the rest of the day. The children were middle-aged and did little physical exercise. All of them – grit your teeth, now – were 'at ideal body weight, lean and muscular, and very healthy'.[7] In fact, their cholesterol level, which by rights should have been sky-high, was barely 60 per cent of normal! These lucky people, without doubt, have a genetic variant (gene for apoprotein B on chromosome 2, it is suspected) which allows them to eat as much as they want without gaining weight. Conversely, we all know people – perhaps you're one – who only have to *look* at a cream cake to start collecting cellulite. Most people lie somewhere between these two extremes.

> Do you feel guilty about leaving leftovers, and eat them – even the rest of the family's – because you don't want to waste the food? The solution is to prepare smaller portions, or learn to be ruthless about throwing food away!

The big news about genes and obesity came when researchers at Rockefeller University in New York City recently reported finding a gene which, if defective, leads to obesity in laboratory mice.[8] (Mice, rats and pigs are commonly used in adiposity research because their metabolisms are considered to resemble those of humans.)

Personally, we dislike research which uses animals as unwilling subjects – the cruelty is often considerable, and one has to wonder how accurately the results can be applied to humans, in any case. In this research, scientists used a strain of mice known as 'obese'. Because of a genetic 'defect' the creature gains up to five times its normal body weight, it often develops insulin-independent diabetes, and it is so poorly equipped to survive that it would die if exposed to the cold because it cannot generate sufficient body heat by burning fat.

Mice have a gene which is 'turned on' in fat tissue, where it appears to produce a hormone-like protein that is secreted by the fat cells into the bloodstream. The theory suggests that this hormone is then carried via the bloodstream to the brain, where it 'communicates' how big or small the fat cells are. The brain can then regulate appetite and eating accordingly. If the gene is defective, as it is in the obese mice, researchers think that it either completely fails to make the appetite-regulating hormone (known as the 'satiety signal') or produces too little of it. Therefore, the brain does not get the proper signal from the fat cells, and the mouse continues to over-eat. Indeed, when obese mice have been injected with this 'satiety signal' (man-ufactured from a normal version of the gene) they have lost weight within a few days. Since the mouse and the human obese genes are 84 per cent identical, researchers (and investors, no doubt) hope that this discovery could soon lead to the devel-opment of a drug that mimics the effect of this hormone.

Shares in one biotech company skyrocketed on Wall Street when the first results of this discovery leaked out. Hardly surprising, considering the size of the potential market, and the fact that 50 million Americans are dieting at any given time.[9] 'Phones started ringing in fat clinics all over the country,' reported the Associated Press when news of the breakthrough was first aired, as thousands of frantic fat people clamoured to be the first human guinea-pigs.[10] 'The potential is astronomical,' exclaimed Dr Arthur Frank, medical director of a George Washington University obesity treatment centre, which was swamped with calls. 'How much would they be willing to pay? You can almost pick a number.' 'The sky's the limit,' agreed Adam Drownowski, a professor of psychiatry who treats eating disorders at the University of Michigan. 'People have been looking for a magic bullet for obesity. And you can bet it is going to be very expensive.'

Expensive – certainly. But . . . things are rarely that easy. Obesity in humans is more complicated than the simple one-gene mouse phenomenon. Indeed, soon after news of the initial research was released, another group of scientists at the Thomas Jefferson University in Pennsylvania declared that in experiments *they* had conducted, it appeared that fat people actually have *higher* levels of the 'ob' hormone than thin people, and they concluded that 'the defect in human obesity lies elsewhere'.[11] Obviously, if fat people have more 'ob' hormone than thin people, it does indicate that the hormone isn't ridding the human body of fat, as it does in mice.

'Obesity in humans is a polygenic condition,' says the lead scientist of the mouse study.[12] In other words, it is the result of small influences from many different genes. He adds that we cannot discount the role of factors such as diet and exercise on human obesity. Indeed not. Other experts agree that our lifestyles continue to play an important – and modifiable – role. Dr Xavier Pi-Sunyer, director of the Obesity Research Center at New York City's St Luke's-Roosevelt Hospital, says only a *fraction* of human obesity is due to a genetic predisposition. The discovery of the mouse gene, he says, 'leaves diet and exercise right where they have always been – central – in preventing obesity.'

> **Canny advertisers know that the stimulus of showing us attractive food can make many of us actually salivate. Knowing this, re-arrange your pantry to keep 'naughty' food out of sight. It'll really help to reduce the pressure on your will-power.**

British scientist Dr Andrew Prentice explains: 'There is an enormous leap from something that works on an obese mouse with a recognized genetic problem and something that works in people – where most obesity has nothing to do with genetic defects.'[13] Dr Prentice, who is head of obesity research at the Medical Research Council's Dunn Nutrition Unit, in Cambridge, estimates that less than 25 per cent of human obesity is due to genetic problems. A recent scientific experiment demonstrated this very convincingly. Conducted at St Luke's-Roosevelt Hospital Center in New York, it studied the food intake of a group of 'diet-resistant' women and men.[14] The doctors measured all the calories these people took in and burned up. They found that their metabolisms were perfectly normal. The real problem was quite clear: they were simply *eating too much. And* they were fooling themselves about how much they ate – they were actually taking in twice as many calories as they believed. To make matters even worse, they were getting a lot less exercise than they believed, too. Commented Dr Steven B. Heymsfield, head of the weight control unit at the hospital: 'These people really cannot invoke some genetic cause as the only explanation for their obesity. The main reason they are overweight is that they are over-eating. Let's not blame it on something that it isn't.'

So yes, genetics certainly has a part to play in the way we respond to our food. But it's not the full story by any means. In particular, don't make the mistake of thinking that you are born to be fat and there's nothing you can do about it. Because there is.

Think for a moment about the huge surge in obesity during the past few years, and common sense will tell you that nothing in our genes could have changed so quickly to make us collectively gain so much weight over such a short period of time. Evolution simply doesn't happen that fast. In fact, in the last 10,000 years (that's right, ten *thousand* years) scientists can only identify a handful of genetic changes in our species. One is the development of the disease sickle-cell anaemia, which was the unfortunate result of a genetic adaptation in some people to protect against the malaria parasite. Another 'recent' change in some adults is their ability to manufacture the enzyme lactase, used by the body to digest the main sugar – lactose – in milk. In all mammals apart from humans, the ability to produce lactase disappears in late childhood, because there is no need for it after weaning. This started to change when humans began domesticating milk-producing animals. Natural selection slowly began to favour those people who retained the genetic ability to manufacture lactase into adulthood: but even so, it is estimated that 75 per cent of adults in all ethnic groups, except those of northwest European origin, still experience lactase deficiency.[15] Another genetic adaptation that has come about in the past 10,000 years is the ability to tolerate gluten, the protein found in

> **Studies show that people who eat infrequently (e.g. one or two large meals daily) put on more weight than people who eat more often. So don't feel guilty about snacking – it can be good for you! But do use the LifePoints system to make sure you're eating high-quality snacks!**

wheat. Apart from these few adaptations – some of which are obviously still under way – very little has changed in our genetic make-up for the past few millennia. Now you can see why it is nonsensical to suggest that the upsurge in obesity over the past decade or two might be primarily a genetic problem. Quite simply, our genes don't change that quickly. Not remotely.

The reason for today's rising tide of plumpness is actually very simple. We're eating the wrong food.

THE NAKED TRUTH ABOUT DIETS

Over the past few years, we've all seen diet crazes come and go. Books are written trumpeting the latest 'breakthroughs' in weight loss, then more books are written 'exposing' the previous books. And so it goes on. Well, here at last is the shocking truth about diets.

- They usually work.
- If you follow a high-fibre, low-fat diet plan – then you'll lose weight.
- If you follow a high-protein, low-carbohydrate diet plan – then you'll lose weight.
- And if you follow a high-fat, low-carbohydrate diet plan – then you'll lose weight, too.

This last one always startles people, because it appears to challenge common sense. But, yes, we did say 'high-fat, low-carbohydrate', and yes, you *can* lose weight very quickly if you eat that sort of diet. We explain why on page 42.

Those are the three main diet combinations. Then there are the 'fringe' diets which gain cult status from time to time, and seem to promise more than just weight loss. Food combining is one such, macrobiotics is another. Most orthodox scientists deride food regimes such as these, on the grounds that the scientific justification advanced for them is incorrect. While that criticism is certainly valid, it's paradoxical that many people do indeed seem to gain very real benefits from these and other 'alternative' diets. Maybe a case for further research?

But even that's not all. There are weirder, even more eccentric diet crazes out there. Eat a popcorn diet, and you'll lose weight. Eat nothing but caviar and champagne, and you'll lose weight. Drink beer all the time, and you'll lose weight. In fact, if you consume almost any kind of bizarre, restricted, unwholesome, risky or lunatic diet, you'll lose weight. You can even lose weight if you count calories, too – but that's a tough one.

> **Make it a rule to always eat at a table. It'll help you resist the temporary craving to snack-out. When the food's on a plate in front of you, you're more aware of what you're actually eating.**

The truth is, virtually every diet ever produced will lead to some weight loss, especially in the first week or two. It's no big deal. The problems – as you may well know from personal experience – are twofold. First: can you keep it up? The answer to this is almost always 'no'. Second: is it good for you? Depending on how bizarre the diet is, the answer is 'probably not', especially over the long term.

The first major scientific survey of the commercial diet industry was published surprisingly recently, in 1993.[16] Readers of *Consumer Reports* (published by the Consumers Union), who had tried to lose weight at least once during the previous three years, were asked to tell about their experiences, and 95,000 of them did so. The results make fascinating reading – and should be *required* reading for anyone thinking about going on a diet! Here's a summary:

- About a quarter of all people who embark on a diet don't need to lose weight! This surprising finding suggests that some of us are simply too anxious to attain a sylph-like figure. Do *you* really need to lose weight? You can find out by following the instructions in 'How to Find Your Body Mass Index' below.
- About a quarter of all dieters are successful in losing weight

and *keeping it off* for two years or so. This still means that 75 per cent fail, but it's a better proposition than the 95 per cent failure rate which is generally quoted (see the Introduction).

- No commercial organization's weight-loss programme was significantly better than any other in helping people to lose weight and keep it off. In fact, you're just as likely to be as successful on your own as you would be paying for (the sometimes very expensive) services and goods offered by these organizations.

- Overall consumer dissatisfaction with weight-loss programmes was higher than that for any other consumer service. Despite their forceful sales pitches, commercial weight-loss organizations often failed to produce scientifically acceptable data on their programmes' results.

How to Find Your Body Mass Index

The Body Mass Index (BMI) is a useful and more reliable guide to body fatness than the old weight and height tables which were popular for many years. Weight in itself is only a very rough guide to the amount of fat that your body contains, and height/weight tables can easily mislead by suggesting that a tall, lean, muscular person is 'overweight', while someone with a small frame but a high percentage of body fat could be rated as 'normal'. The BMI has been found to be an altogether more accurate reflection of body fatness, and is not excessively biased by variations in height.[17] Here's an easy way to work out what your BMI is:

Using a calculator, multiply your height in metres by itself. Write down the result. Press the 'clear' button on your calculator and enter your weight in kilograms. Press the 'divide' button then enter the number you've just written down.

Press the 'equals' button to learn what your BMI is. Now rate yourself:[18]

Your BMI	Classification
Less than 20	underweight
20–25	desirable range
25–30	overweight
30 or more	obese

ARE YOU AN APPLE OR A PEAR?

Where do you carry your excess baggage? Recently, scientists have found that your individual shape – apple or pear – can be an important factor in predicting your future health. People who carry excess weight above their waistline are apple-shaped, those whose weight settles around the hips and buttocks are shaped like pears. Most overweight men tend to be apple-shaped (think of the classic beer belly), while most women are pears.

Furthermore, apples are much more prone to heart disease than pears. In fact, many scientists now believe that the body shape can predict cardiovascular disease better than the actual amount of obesity. This may be because abdominal fat is more metabolically active than below-the-waist fat, and is associated with insulin resistance (a precursor to diabetes). It may also be a cause of high blood pressure. For women, research indicates that apples are less fertile than pears. One study suggests that pear-shaped women have higher levels of HDL, the 'good' cholesterol associated with a lower risk of heart disease. Another study finds that pear-shaped women are less likely to develop breast cancer. To find out what shape you are, calculate your waist-to-hip ratio as follows:

1) With a tape measure, measure your waist at its *narrowest* point when your stomach is relaxed:

   Waist: inches

   ---

2) Measure your hips at their *widest* (where your bottom sticks out the most):

   Hips: inches

   ---

3) Now divide your waist measurement by your hip measurement:

   Waist ÷ hip =   waist-to-hip ratio

The higher the waist-to-hip ratio, the more apple-shaped your figure. If the result is 0.75 or less – smile, – you're a pear! If it's 0.75 to 0.8, you're a mini-apple, but if it's over 0.8 then you're a Cox's orange pippin! For men, the risk of serious obesity-related diseases rises above a waist-to-hip ratio of 0.95; for women, the cut off point is 0.8. Your body will tend to use up fat which has been most recently stored, so if necessary you may be able to turn yourself back from an apple into a pear. Try taking this test again in about two months – you'll find it very encouraging!

CHECK IN HERE FOR THE LIFEPOINTS DIET!

If it's true that only one in four diets eventually work, we want to give you every possible chance of being in that top 25 per cent! In order to do that, you have to be realistic about your change of lifestyle, because that is the *only way* you're going to achieve any worthwhile, long-term progress. There's an old saying that 'Success by the inch is a cinch – by the yard, it's hard.' Remember that motto well – because it's going to be a key article of faith in the LifePoints Diet. Time and time again, people have shed near-miraculous amounts of weight, only to regain it all – and more besides – when they stop dieting.

> **Most people don't drink enough fluid. Dieters in particular should avoid the physical stress that dehydration can cause, so make a point of drinking about 6–8 glasses of water a day.**

Persistent weight regain after dieting – it's called the 'yo-yo' effect – is dangerous. Research shows that people who do this have a higher incidence of heart disease and diabetes than those who never diet.[19] As Professor Dean Ornish, director of the Preventive Medicine Research Institute in Sausalito, explains: 'When you over-eat, your fat cells grow larger. If you keep over-eating, you begin forming new fat cells. You also gain weight. The size of your fat cells may decrease if you restrict food intake for a while, but the number does not. When you first lose weight by restricting the amount of food you eat, you lose both muscle and fat tissue. But when you gain weight back, you regain proportionately more fat than you lost.' That's the theory, and it's been proven over and over again in practice. In a recent Dutch study, men who experienced many life events in a short period of time showed a marked weight gain (losing your job, getting divorced, having children and other major upheavals often generate weight fluctuations).[20] A year later this weight gain had disappeared in almost all subgroups of these men. The exception was the subgroup that tried to lose weight by dieting; those who dieted *gained yet more weight.*[21]

We say the LifePoints Diet is for life. This *doesn't* mean that you're going to have to survive on a restricted food intake for the rest of your life. It *does* mean that the changes you're going to make to your eating habits – although small individually – together amount to an impressive, long-term lifestyle improvement. While you'll certainly experience some useful and encouraging short-term results, that really isn't the point. Think of it as a re-education for your tastebuds. Our aim is to help you experience food as it was meant to be: delicious, irresistible but also nourishing and health-giving *for a lifetime.* Within a few weeks of starting the LifePoints Diet, it will seem like second nature to you. That's because the principles behind it are entirely natural. Remember: 'Success by the inch is a cinch – by the yard, it's hard!'

> **Don't be tempted to think that just skipping a meal a day is an easy way to lose weight – it's not! Grazing (eating 4–6 small meals throughout the day) has been shown to be a more effective way of keeping your body supplied with just enough energy to avoid those dangerous peaks and troughs which so often lead to bingeing.**

Let's start the LifePoints Diet right now – get out a pen and do the LifePoints Check-In. The following seven guidelines lay down the basic principles for the weeks ahead. But guidelines without commitment mean nothing! Now, it's your turn to read them and make them *yours* by filling in the statements which follow.

1 Wise Up and Size Up!

What's *your* motivation for dieting? Is it to fit into a dress or swimsuit? Or is it to become a healthy, active person? People who are motivated to lose weight for short-term reasons are generally not as successful as those who attempt to lose weight because they genuinely desire to be healthier, more active people.

I want to lose weight because:

_____

2 Arrest the Stress!

Have you recently: moved, broken off a relationship, or under-gone work-related changes? Are you feeling lonely or bored? Trying to change your eating habits when you're in the throes of a highly stressful situation isn't advised. Stress often leads to an urge to over-eat, which means the chances of failure are increased, and this will be de-motivating for you.

What sources of stress do I have in my life now?

_____

Which of these sometimes cause me to over-eat?

_____

Which of these could interfere with my success at losing weight?

_____

What practical steps can I take to reduce these stress factors – and increase my success with the LifePoints Diet?

_____

3 Screen Your Team!

One of the great secret weapons to help you cope with the changes that lie ahead is to create a small team of sympathetic, supportive friends. People who are going to lend an ear when necessary, and who will be entirely positive about your efforts. Let them read the LifePoints books so they understand this system and its unique approach. Maybe one or two of them might even join you! Choose friends with whom you feel comfortable and who can motivate you. Communicate often with them.

The members of my LifePoints team are:

_____

4 Slim to Win!

Many people fail to understand how important it is to set goals for themselves. Others do set goals, but make them hopelessly unrealistic. Some people feel they won't be 'worthwhile' or 'beautiful' unless they weigh a certain amount or wear a certain size. This doesn't encourage a positive self-image, nor is it a realistic tool to help you lose weight. The two most important things to remember about goal-setting are: 1) to make your goals realistic and 2) not to turn aside until you've achieved them.

Give some thought now to the precise goals you're going to set. If you intend to set a specific goal for weight loss (pounds or kilos lost) then do it in stages. For example: let's imagine you initially lose 5 pounds. Now, if you've set this as your goal, you'll feel proud, positive and motivated to continue. But if you've set an impossibly high target – say, 30 pounds – then you could easily feel downhearted. Remember – 'success by the inch is a cinch – by the yard, it's hard!'

> **Study after study indicates that the slower you lose weight, the more likely you are to lose fat rather than muscle tissue. Also, slower weight loss is more likely to be kept off permanently! So aim to lose no more than 1 per cent of your body weight a week . . . ½ to 1 pound a week is about right for many people.**

But weight isn't the only yardstick you can use to set a personal goal. Other possible targets might include: How well do your clothes fit? Can you 'pinch an inch' of fat at your waistline or at the back of your arm? When you jump up and down in front of a full-length mirror, nude, does anything jiggle that shouldn't? How do you feel – energetic or wiped out? Do you have good muscle tone, or are you flabby? Are you able to walk up a few flights of stairs without panting? When you put your hand on your thigh or hip, do you feel muscle or fat? Any of these targets can be used, if appropriate for you, to serve both as a goal and as a way of monitoring the progress you're making.

Should you aim to achieve your weight loss goal over a given period of time? We don't think so. The LifePoints Diet *isn't* a 'crash' diet. A crash produces a casualty, and a crash diet produces a casualty, too – you! Let those pounds melt away in their own time. You'll be surprised how quickly it happens!

My primary weight-loss goal is:

_____

> **There's no need to weigh yourself every day. Everyone experiences small fluctuations in weight – small increases may discourage you, deterring you from healthy eating habits. Establish a regular schedule for weighing; once every week is often enough. Pay more attention to how fit you feel, rather than what the scales say.**

5 Commit to Fit

Gentle, invigorating exercise is an integral part of the Life-Points Diet. In our experience, people often try to ignore this aspect, or just skip it entirely. Please don't! Becoming more active is one of the most important things you can do when losing weight. It can make you feel good, improve self-esteem, and give you more energy. It also helps to build strength and endurance while it conditions your heart. And exercise has been shown to be a major predictor of success at maintaining a weight loss. You don't have to be a triathlete or marathon runner to exercise . . . just follow our suggestions!

I agree to increase my physical activity: (write YES and sign it!)

_____

6 WRITE YOUR BITES!

At the back of this book you'll find a blank LifePoints Daily Planner form which we'd like you to use. Photocopy several of them and carry them with you, in your personal organizer or bag. We want you to use these forms to keep a running check on your progress. But that's not all – you can go further and keep a food diary, which also keeps a record of emotions that may trigger your eating, such as loneliness, boredom, anger, frustration or simply watching television (all those food commercials!). You can also use this to keep track of exercise and your mood while eating. Keeping a record helps you to understand how and why you eat, and has proven to be an important part of habit change. Food records can also be of great help to professionals (e.g. dieticians) in identifying situations or foods which are problem areas that need working on. Keeping a food diary can help you gain control over these situations, ultimately leading to healthier eating habits.

I agree to keep a faithful and regular daily record of all the food I eat (write YES and sign it!)

7 CEASE THE GREASE!

As you'll see, the LifePoints Diet is probably lower in fat than the diet you're used to. Most people eat far too much fat these days, and you can see the unfortunate consequences everywhere you look. Surging rates of obesity, high cholesterol, heart disease and breast, colon, rectal and prostate cancers are all directly related to the amount of fat we consume. Experts estimate that an unhealthy 40 per cent of the average Westerner's calorie intake comes from fat, but in our experience many people consume considerably more than this.[22] Reducing

> **Men almost always lose weight much more easily than women, probably because they have more muscle tissue to raise metabolism. Unfortunately, that's the way the cookie crumbles. But it doesn't mean that if you can do it, he can too!**

the fat you consume on the LifePoints Diet is not as difficult as you might fear, but it does involve some initial dietary adjustments.

The *good* news is that once you've become used to lower-fat fare, you'll find high-fat foods greasy and objectionable! As Professor Kan Stanfill from the University of Oklahoma Health Sciences Center explains: 'One of the most important things to remember is that your taste perception will change as you continue decreasing the fat. It can take anywhere from six to eight weeks for an individual to become accustomed to a lower-fat diet and to find it as fully satisfying, from a taste standpoint, as a higher-fat diet.'[23] Right now, we want you to do two things. First, take the quiz that follows (answer honestly!) to find out what percentage of your current diet consists of fat. You may be in for a surprise! Then, we want you to commit to reducing your fat intake – using the techniques and recipes you'll find in this book and others in the LifePoints series.

I agree to reduce my fat intake by following the LifePoints system, and I'm prepared to keep on going for a few weeks while my tastebuds make the change (write YES and sign it!)

_____

AND NOW – DO THE FAT CHECK!

This simple quiz will probably amaze you! Devised by clever researchers at Seattle's Fred Hutchinson Cancer Research Center, it is designed to estimate quickly the percentage of fat in your total dietary intake of calories. You don't need to refer to anything like a food diary, so you can do it right now!

Here's how to do it. Think about your diet over the past three months and answer each of the following questions with a number from the list below. If a question doesn't apply to your diet, leave it blank. (For instance, if you don't eat red meat, don't answer questions 5, 6 and 19 – your score is based on the rest of your diet.)

1 = Always
2 = Often
3 = Occasionally
4 = Rarely or Never

	In the past three months, when you . . .	Your answer 1 to 4
1	Ate fish, did you avoid frying it?	
2	Ate chicken, did you avoid frying it?	
3	Ate chicken, did you remove the skin?	
4	Ate spaghetti or noodles, did you eat it plain or with a meatless tomato sauce?	
5	Ate red meat, did you trim all the visible fat?	
6	Ate ground beef, did you choose extra lean?	
7	Ate bread, rolls or muffins, did you eat them without butter or margarine?	
8	Drank milk, was it skimmed milk instead of whole milk?	
9	Ate cheese, was it a reduced-fat variety?	
10	Ate a frozen dessert, was it sorbet, ice milk, or a non-fat yogurt or ice cream?	
11	Ate cooked vegetables, did you eat them without adding butter, margarine, salt pork or bacon fat?	
12	Ate cooked vegetables, did you avoid frying them?	
13	Ate potatoes, were they cooked by a method other than frying?	
14	Ate boiled or baked potatoes, did you eat them without butter, margarine or sour cream?	
15	Ate green salads with dressing, did you use a low-fat or non-fat dressing?	
16	Ate a dessert, did you eat only fruit?	

17	Ate a snack, was it raw vegetables?	
18	Ate a snack, was it fresh fruit?	
19	Cooked red meat, did you trim all the fat before cooking?	
20	Used mayonnaise or a mayonnaise-type dressing, was it low-fat or non-fat?	

Now it's time to learn the truth! First, transfer the numbers above to the score sheet below. Disregard questions that were left blank. You'll see that the items are arranged within five fat-lowering strategies rather than according to their order in the quiz. Add up the total for each strategy, then whip out your calculator and follow the instructions.

Strategy 1: How well do you avoid frying your food?

Question 1 _____

Question 2 _____

Question 12 _____

Question 13 _____

Subtotal _____

Now divide by 4 to learn your average: _____

Strategy 2: How well do you avoid fatty meat?

Question 3 _____

Question 5 _____

Question 6 _____

Question 19 _____

Subtotal _____

Now divide by 4 to learn your average: _____

Strategy 3: How well do you avoid fat as a flavouring?

Question 4 _____

Question 7 _____

Question 11 _____

Question 14 _____

Subtotal _____

Now divide by 4 to learn your average: _____

Strategy 4: How well do you substitute low-fat or non-fat versions of foods?

Question 8 _____

Question 9 _____

Question 10 _____

Question 15 _____

Question 20 _____

Subtotal _____

Now divide by 5 to learn your average: _____

Strategy 5: How well do you replace fatty foods with fresh produce?

Question 16 _____

Question 17 _____

Question 18 _____

Subtotal _____

Now divide by 3 to learn your average: _____

Now add up all your averages and write the grand total here _____. Lastly, divide this figure by 5 to calculate your overall score, and write it here _____. Then check the chart below:

If your overall average is	Your percentage of fat from calories is
1.0 to 1.5	under 25%
1.5 to 2	25 to 29%
2 to 2.5	30 to 34%
2.5 to 3	35 to 39%
3 to 3.5	40 to 44%
3.5 to 4	45% or more

Make sure you take the Fat Check again when you've completed your first month on the LifePoints Diet!

LIFEPOINTS – BEYOND CALORIE-COUNTING

There is now substantial, compelling and unambiguous scientific evidence to demonstrate that the traditional concept of weight loss by counting calories is – for most practical purposes – utterly useless. We have already seen how anything from 75 to 95 per cent of calorie-counting diets fail. If calorie-restricted diets really worked, then there would be few people in the Western world with an obesity problem. The fact that Westerners are today far fatter than ever before – and yet consume *fewer* calories than they did at the turn of the 20th century – tells us all we need to know about the usefulness of calories as a means of controlling weight.[24]

For many people, counting calories is still the only 'correct' way to shed pounds (despite overwhelming evidence of failure). Some people even believe – quite incorrectly – that a low-calorie food is the same thing as a healthy food! These myths – because that's what they are – die very, very slowly. Try this quick quiz to discover how many calorie myths you still swallow. You may get a surprise!

1) You're trying to decide which is the least fattening of two foods on the menu. They both have the same calorie count. Which one do you decide to pick?

a) Flip a coin – since both foods have the same number of calories, it doesn't matter.

b) The one that gets most of its calories from fat.

c) The one that gets most of its calories from carbohydrate.

2) When scientists analyse a food to measure its calorie content, what colour are the calories they finally extract?

a) Light pink

b) No colour

c) Grey

3) Which one of the following statements defines what a calorie is?

a) The amount of heat energy required to raise the temperature of 1 gram of water from 14.5°C to 15.5°C.

b) 4.184 watt-seconds, or joules.

c) The amount of food which makes the average human put on 1 gram of weight.

4) How many calories do you use up if you run vigorously for one minute?

a) 15

b) 150

c) 15,000

5) Calories can be divided into 'good calories' and 'bad calories'.

a) Yes

b) No

c) Maybe

Now check your answers. For question 1, the conventional view of nutrition would state that answer (a) is the right one. Early in the 20th century, scientists demonstrated that many animals could produce body fat from a diet which was naturally high in carbohydrate.[25] It was also known that animals who hibernated – and therefore needed to increase their fat stores drastically before the winter's sleep – could fatten themselves very effectively on a high-carbohydrate diet.[26] On the basis of evidence such as this, most scientists, doctors and the population at large came to believe that carbohydrate-rich food was the most fattening. In point of fact, the very reverse is true. As scientists established several decades ago, the human body's highly complex metabolic processes handle fat, carbohydrate and protein in very different ways to those of the hibernating or laboratory animal. By doing studies on people – not animals – scientists now know the truth. When you eat a meal which is high in carbohydrate, the body has to work very hard indeed to convert those calories into bodily fat. Think about it: to transform a baked potato (high carbohydrate, low fat) into additional fat on your waistline, some highly complicated physiological processes have to go on. Those processes consume energy – lots of it – to the extent that a quarter of the calories in a high-carbohydrate foodstuff are consumed in the effort to turn that baked potato into body fat.[27] Because this process is so inefficient, the body really doesn't favour turning carbohydrate into fat – it's too much hard work! In fact, a mere 1 per cent of the carbohydrates we normally eat in our diets usually get turned into fat.[28]

Now let's dump a large wad of butter onto that baked potato. Suddenly, it's become a high-fat food. Danger! Now things look very different. Turning a fatty food into fat on the waistline presents no major problems – dietary fat is the only nutrient that can beat a direct path to the body's fat depots![29] In this case, the energy consumed by the process is very low – in fact, only 3 per cent of the food's calories will be used up.[30]

Don't worry if your rate of weight loss slows down or stops from time to time. If you hit a 'plateau' like this, don't cut back on your food intake – your body will think you're in a starvation situation! Stick to the same food intake, but perhaps gently increase your exercise schedule, and you'll find weight loss will resume.

The right answer to question 1 is therefore option (c) – given two foods with similar calorie yields, the carbohydrate-rich food will be considerably less fattening. Simply switching from a high-fat diet to one high in carbohydrates will result in painless net calorie loss to your body – *without having to reduce your total calorie intake*. The LifePoints diet takes full advantage of this important phenomenon.

How did you answer question 2? Sorry, but it's a trick question, of course. Part of the confusion which surrounds calories – and there's lots of it – revolves around the definition of the calorie itself. In order to understand calories, you need to remember this important fact: calories have no tangible existence on their own. You can't see them, you can't taste them, and you certainly can't separate them out from the food itself. That fact makes them very different from other nutrients found in food, such as vitamin C. Give an orange to a biochemist, and after some chemical sorcery in the lab she'll be able to give you a test-tube containing most of that orange's vitamin C. Not so with calories! In Latin, 'calor' means 'heat', and that gives us a clue to the real function of the calorie. It is simply the name of a unit used to measure heat energy. A food's calorie number tells you how much energy is locked up inside the food. It *doesn't* tell you what the food contains, nor how good the food is for you, nor how much of that energy will go to your fat stores if you eat the food. Correct answer: (b).

The right answer to number 3 is . . . sorry, another trick question! Both (a) and (b) are correct. The really useful answer would have been (c) but, as we've seen, calories do not measure how much weight a food is going to make you put on. Scientists have conventionally used a laboratory instrument called a 'bomb calorimeter' to measure the calorie yield of a food. They take a portion of the food in question – say a slice of cheesecake – and seal it inside a container. The air is pumped out and oxygen gas is pumped in. Then, an electric spark ignites the oxygen and – bang! – the food combusts, and heat energy is released. The container is immersed in a water bath, and by measuring the rise in the water's temperature it is possible to calculate the calorie yield of the food. If you're thinking that this technique doesn't sound much like the human digestive system, you're absolutely right. Although humans have an astoundingly large surface area of digestive tract through which the nutrients in foods are absorbed – if you spread it out it would be larger than a tennis court – we don't absorb *all* the nutrients in food, and we don't use *all* the potential heat energy locked up in foodstuffs. Real world systems, such as digestion, are always far more complex than lab models.

As if all this wasn't difficult enough, question 4 highlights some additional calorie confusion. The right answer is (c). You may be surprised (overjoyed!) to learn that you can use up 15,000 calories a minute while running, but don't get too excited! A 'calorie' when popularly used in connection with food usually means a 'kilocalorie', or 1000 calories. Sometimes you'll see it written like this: 'kcal', sometimes like this: 'Cal', but most often, just plain old 'calorie'. So, yes, it is scientifically correct to say that you can use up 15,000 calories a minute by running, but in terms most of us understand, this actually means 15 kilocalories, usually shortened to 15 calories. Which is about the calorie yield of half a carrot.

> **Although it may appear attractive, fasting is not a good way to lose weight. Prolonged fasts can cause serious harm by depleting the levels of protein, calcium, phosphorus, sodium and potassium in your body. Also, the LifePoints Diet is all about finding a new, better and permanent way of eating. It's not a quick fix!**

If you've read a few diet books or magazine articles on the subject, you'll know that exercise by itself can't burn up very many calories. Walk briskly for an hour and you'll burn off 360 calories (one milkshake). Cycle for the same time and you'll use 400 calories (a scoop of rich ice cream). Swim and you'll disperse 525 calories (2 cups of chick peas). Based on these sums, traditional dietary theory declares that you're obviously not going to get thin just by going for the burn! That's true, as far as it goes. However, a gentle exercise programme can indeed help us in the weight reduction process, and it is an important part of the LifePoints Diet. If you've always been allergic to exercise programmes, *don't* stop reading! We have something new and very pleasurable to offer you, as you'll see in the next chapter. We're going to use exercise to increase your basal metabolic rate, meaning that your body will start to burn more fat even when you're doing nothing at all! Exercise plays a critical role not only in burning fat, but also in our longer-term goal of keeping weight off. You're going to surprise yourself . . . we promise!

The right answer to question five is (b). There are no such things as 'good' calories or 'bad' calories. Although various books and weight-reduction programmes may try to claim otherwise, scientifically speaking a calorie is a calorie is a calorie (i.e. a unit of measurement). Pretending that there are different 'types' of calorie, or that some calories can magically burn off those excess pounds, is scientific bunkum, and only makes an already confused area even more chaotic. This, too, serves to illustrate yet another major shortcoming with calorie-counting: it does not discriminate between good food and bad. When you decide your diet on the sole criterion of a food's calorie yield, you run the very real risk of excluding nourishing foods, while including foods which are low calorie – but low on nutrition, too.

> **People often have very fixed views on whether they should or shouldn't take a combined vitamin/mineral pill while they're trying to lose weight. Unlike most other dietary regimes, the LifePoints Diet is designed to provide you with a naturally excellent intake of vitamins and minerals. Even so, we still believe that a good food supplement is worthwhile 'nutritional insurance'. But everyone to their own!**

When you start a low-calorie diet, your body assumes that you're starving – because as far as your body is concerned, dieting and starving are one and the same thing. Initially, you will certainly lose weight. But starvation is a life-threatening event and, cleverly, you already have an excellent survival strategy lined up for just such a situation, ready to be implemented at the drop of a calorie. The first thing to happen is that your metabolic rate lowers in order to conserve energy. The longer your food intake continues to be below what it expects, the harder your body tries to preserve that precious energy locked up as fat. That's why the first week of any diet produces an impressive result, yet subsequent weeks often achieve little, if anything. Low-calorie diets are doomed to failure, because your body's deep-rooted instincts are fighting you all the way. And sooner or later, they'll win – intelligence always loses to instinct!

One notorious way in which your instincts overwhelm your rational mind is through the binge impulse. You will surely be familiar with it – a few days into the diet, and things are looking good. Then, in one insane and unrestrained moment, you find yourself behaving like a great white shark in a crowded swimming pool. Eat! Eat! Eat! As you frantically succumb to the urge to devour anything that could possibly have a calorie or two associated with it, you start to feel helpless and guilty. How could you be so weak? How could you have ruined all your hard work in a momentary feeding frenzy? This sort of negative innertalk can even lead to serious eating disorders such as bulimia. Our message to you is: take it easy on yourself! Your poor old body is just trying to do what it thinks is best for you. In fact, the binge impulse is a hugely successful survival strategy. When faced with a severe food shortage, your instincts become supersensitive to any potential source of food – and, of course, in today's society there are *unlimited* sources of food available everywhere. Drop your guard for just one instant, and the ancient survival instincts take over. Now you can begin to see how significantly different the LifePoints Diet is to conventional calorie-counting. We aim to work *with* your instincts, not ineffectually oppose them. We want them to protect you as they're supposed to, and not relentlessly challenge your willpower. Because that's the only way we're going to achieve longterm success.

Sometimes we jokingly say that low-calorie diets should be banned on the grounds that they constitute cruel and unusual punishment. Just look at some of the problems associated with this form of weight reduction, and you'll wonder how even a hero (or heroine) would ever attempt it:

- Most calorie-restricted diets reduce the calorie count simply by cutting food portion sizes. This does nothing to retrain your food perceptions, and demands super-human discipline (or a strong streak of masochism) to stick to
- Along with this, you feel hungry most of the time (and that's just downright miserable) leading to . . .
- Depression
- Bloating and distended stomach
- Constipation
- Feeling cold all the time
- Hair loss
- Headaches
- Lack of energy
- Low blood pressure leading to dizziness
- Sleep disruption
- Failure to produce collagen, the major protein of all connective tissues
- Loss of lean tissue
- Menstrual difficulties
- Water retention
- Yeast infections.

The final nail in the coffin of low-calorie diets must surely be the abundant evidence of rebound obesity, sometimes called the 'yo-yo' effect. The Dutch study into rebound obesity (referred to on page 20) makes no sense to those who believe weight gain is a 'calorie problem', and therefore weight loss can be accomplished simply by restricting calories. But when you see it in terms of a survival strategy, it makes perfect sense: those men had already been through a number of stressful life events, and the threat of starvation (i.e. dieting) seemed, to their bodies, to be just one more hazard. Their bodies actually responded splendidly by trying to conserve every last calorie.

In fact, many scientific studies now confirm that if you want to put on weight, one of the best ways to do it is to diet. Weight gain is particularly provoked by 'diet cycling' (continual diet/binge cycles), and it is such a well-accepted phenomenon that it is sometimes used in a clinical situation to help underweight patients put on bulk. How, precisely, does this happen? It's probably connected to the production of an enzyme called

> **If you eat out a lot, you'll find the LifePoints Listing very helpful. Many restaurant or snack-bar foods are basically high-LifePoints, low-RiskPoints foods, but are then spoilt by the addition of sauces, dressings and other 'invisible' naughties. With a small amount of tweaking (tomato sauce instead of cream on your pasta) you can eat well!**

lipoprotein lipase (LPL) which is responsible for storing bodily fat. After starting a diet, LPL levels initially drop, then remorselessly rise again – sometimes to 25 times the normal level. The fatter you are to begin with, the more LPL you'll produce when dieting.

To summarize: If calorie-restricted diets worked effectively, then there would be few people in the Western world with an obesity problem. But it doesn't – and sadly there are. For realistic weight control purposes, calorie-counting is now dead.

LifePoints – Beyond Counting Fat

Because calorie-counting has consistently failed so many of us, people have started to look for other ways to guide them through their food choices. One of the more recent methods is to restrict the number of grams of fat in the food you eat. Fat – and in particular saturated fat (mainly from animal sources) – is without doubt our number one dietary enemy today. So reducing the amount of fat you consume is an excellent idea, and is an important part of the LifePoints Diet. Since fat is by far the biggest source of calories in your diet, decreasing your fat consumption will invariably reduce your calorie intake. And counting grams of fat (unlike counting calories) doesn't require a calculator or a brain like Einstein's. Furthermore, by reducing or eliminating those foods which are high in fat, you are starting to make some sensible judgements about the comparative worth of various foods in your diet – something which mere calorie-counting cannot help you do.

There are really only two significant problems with counting fat. First, scientific evidence has shown for many years that certain types of fat – principally the saturated fatty acids – have an especially unhealthy impact on our lives. Unfortunately, simply knowing the total amount of fat in a food won't tell you how much saturated fat it contains. And keeping running totals of your *total* fat intake, your *saturated* fat intake, and then calculating (say) how many more grams of fat – but not saturated fat – you're allowed during the day is far too complicated for most of us mortals.

> **Do you taste your food – *really* taste it – or just gulp it down? Think about this the next time you eat. Try timing yourself – if it takes less than ten seconds to demolish each morsel, you're speeding! When you consciously relax into a less tense eating pattern, you'll magically find that any urge to over-eat also diminishes.**

Fortunately, the LifePoints Diet can come to the rescue here. Each food in our ratings system has two numbers – its LifePoints rating and its Risk-Points rating. The LifePoints number tells you about the beneficial nutrients in the food, the RiskPoints number tells you about the less healthy elements. The beauty of the Risk-Points number is this: it can help you to achieve *two* important goals with regard to fat. To begin with, it ensures that your *total* fat consumption remains healthily low. How low? Well, if your RiskPoints daily total adds up to no more than 100, you'll have eaten no more than 40 grams of fat. For the average woman, whose energy intake comes to about 2200 calories, that represents about 16 per cent of calories. For a man, consuming about 2,900 calories, it keeps your total fat intake down to about 12 per cent of calories. These are the kinds of levels which, research shows, our species has naturally consumed for most of our history.

In many parts of the world – China, for example – people still consume this level of fat in their diets. The result? Many of the 'diseases of civilization' which so plague us in the West are virtually unknown. Why do we suggest you keep your fat intake down to this level? Here's how *The New York Times* put it when reporting the results of the largest ever scientific study into the diets and health of the Chinese people: 'Reducing dietary fat to less than 30 per cent of calories, as is currently recommended for Americans, may not be enough to curb the risk of heart disease and cancer. To make a significant impact, the Chinese data imply, a maximum of 20 per cent of calories from fat – and preferably only 10 to 15 per cent – should be consumed.'[31]

The China Study is a landmark in the science of epidemiology. It began in 1983, with the aim of exploring the dietary causes of cancer. Since then, it has been expanded to include heart, metabolic and infectious diseases. And these findings are only the beginning. Dr T. Colin Campbell, a nutritional biochemist from Cornell University and the American mastermind of the study, predicts that this 'living laboratory' will continue to generate vital findings for the next 40 to 50 years.

A naturally low-fat diet can do many remarkable things beyond helping with weight loss. Perhaps the most wonderful – still largely unrecognized – is its ability, in some people, to break down the plaques which build up and eventually block coronary arteries . . . we're talking about nothing less than reversing heart disease! Amongst other benefits, increased flow of blood in these arteries can also appreciably reduce the pain of angina.[32]

> **The China Study has confirmed that obesity is clearly related to *what* you eat, rather than how much. The Chinese actually consume 20 per cent *more* calories than Westerners, but Westerners are 25 per cent fatter! The reason is that fat in our diet.**

So by keeping your Risk-Points to no more than 100, you'll be enjoying a naturally low-fat diet. But here the RiskPoints number is doubly clever. Because not only does it keep a check on your total fat intake, it also intelligently guides you *away* from food which is unhealthily high in saturated fat, and steers you *towards* food which is low in it. Saturated fat is irrefutably linked to the development of coronary heart disease, and probably to certain cancers too. Until recently, it was thought that all types of fat were equally fattening for humans (they all yield the same number of calories). However, a growing body of scientific evidence now points to the fact that saturated fat is especially bad for slimmers. For example, while unsaturated fats can inhibit the body's creation of fat from carbohydrates, saturated fat does not.[33] Further, the body seems to prefer to burn unsaturated fat in preference to saturated fat, which it finds easier to place in storage in fat cells.[34] For all these good reasons, we don't want you getting all your fat intake as unhealthy saturated fat. And here, you can think of this aspect of the RiskPoints equation as a silent friend always present in the background – gently nudging you away from unhealthy foods and leading you to the healthier choices. You may not notice it, but it's there, working for you all the time!

> **The LifePoints Diet is not about self-denial, it's about enjoying your food – and feeling good about yourself afterwards. If you really find you can't relish a meal without huge helpings of high-fat foods, try stoking up on any *fresh* food with a high LifePoints number before your main meal. You'll find this will significantly diminish your appetite for fats.**

The second significant problem with simply counting the number of grams of fat in food concerns all the nutrients that you're *not* counting when you count fat. Knowing that a particular food may be high in fat is useful, because it helps you to avoid it. But it doesn't help you to choose *good* food!

Avoiding unhealthy food is only half of the secret of planning a good diet. The other half is knowing which food you *should* choose. And here, counting fat won't help you – but the LifePoints Diet will. Specifically, each food has a LifePoints number which judges its overall content of essential nutrients. The higher the LifePoints number, the better. Simple, isn't it?

To summarize: knowing the amount of fat in a foodstuff is a useful first step towards planning a healthy, weight-reducing diet. The LifePoints Diet goes beyond this first step by discriminating between various types of fat, and by positively guiding you towards the healthiest food choices.

Fast Facts About Fat

The whole area of dietary fat is one of the most confusing for many people. Here, we give answers to the most common questions people ask us . . .

What does 'fat-free' mean on a food label?
It *should* mean precisely what it says – zero fat. However, watch out for some cheating! If a product says '85 per cent fat free' it may mean that the product is actually 15 per cent fat by weight. Big difference! 15 grams of fat per 100 grams of food means that fully 40 per cent of that food's calorie yield could be supplied by fat. This mathematical mendacity is one reason why we suggest you use the RiskPoints number – it's far simpler, and it provides a uniform basis for you to make comparisons.

What are trans fatty acids?
Trans fatty acids occur when vegetable or fish oils have hydrogen bubbled through them to make them more solid (hydrogenation). The resulting fat can be used in a semi-solid spread like margarine, to prolong the shelf life of baked goods such as biscuits, and for deep frying. Increasingly, researchers suspect that trans fat may be nearly as bad for humans as saturated fat. Prudent advice would therefore be to avoid or minimize use of products whose major ingredients include 'partially hydrogenated vegetable oils'. Remember that the RiskPoints number will automatically steer you away from high-fat foods, and from saturated fats, but it won't currently warn you off food which contains trans fats. This may change in future LifePoints publications.

What are essential fatty acids?
The two classes of essential fatty acids (EFAs) are named omega-6 and omega-3. Both are necessary for good health and, through a complicated transformation process, they become biologically active in many of the body's metabolic systems. They are called 'essential'

because the body cannot make them, and therefore they must be obtained from food sources. Omega-6 fatty acids (e.g. linoleic acid) are found in vegetable seeds and the oils produced from them. Good sources include oils made from safflower, sunflower, corn, soya, evening primrose, pumpkin, walnut and wheat germ. Omega-3 fatty acids (e.g. alpha linolenic acid) are found in deep-water fish oils, linseed, rapeseed (canola) and soya bean oil. Even people who consume high-fat diets may be low on essential fatty acids, because they're simply not eating foods which contain them. So don't feel guilty if you sometimes snack on modest amounts of nuts and seeds, and do try to use these oils cold-pressed – heating will reduce or destroy their EFA content.

I've heard that you can lose weight on a high-fat diet.
What you've heard is true! It astonishes many people when they learn that a very high-fat diet will induce weight loss, but it certainly will – and quickly. Here's how: blood glucose is the primary source of energy in animals, and is normally manufactured by your body from the carbohydrates in your diet. For storage purposes, glucose is converted to glycogen and then stored in the liver, muscles and fat. If you eliminate all dietary carbohydrates, and only eat foods which contain fat and protein, what will your body do? Well, with its main source of energy gone, your body is forced to burn fat – both dietary and bodily – as its primary fuel. You may think this sounds highly unnatural, and indeed it is. Nature never meant us to obtain our energy this way. When body fats are broken down to provide energy, toxic levels of compounds known as ketones (chemicals related to acetone) are produced, creating acidity, irritating the kidneys and allowing your blood sugar level to plummet. This isn't slimming, it's chemical warfare against your own body. Emphatically not advised.

What do you think of the new fat substitutes?
We take a pragmatic view of the new generation of fake fats coming onto the market, and say that they may well

be of use – to *some* people. Can they help you reduce your fat consumption? Yes, without a doubt. Will they help you retrain your tastebuds to favour fresher, less fatty food? No, not at all. You decide!

LIFEPOINTS – BEYOND THE GLYCAEMIC INDEX

The glycaemic index made headlines recently when a spate of books on the subject of 'insulin resistance' were published. In America, where the media likes nothing more than dishing the dirt on the latest healthy-food-turned-villain, *The New York Times* printed an article based on this theory, which suggested that 'Eating Pasta Makes You Fat'. Many other newspapers and TV news shows picked up the story, and even embellished it. One newspaper reported: 'Contrary to current thinking, high-carbohydrate/low-fat diets are "absolutely killing us."'[35] Shocking! But what's it all about? Stories such as these – and they appear quite regularly – are often a mixture of facts, hypotheses, hype and distortions. At the heart of this particular story lies a modest little number known as the glycaemic index, which might indeed prove useful to some people. So let's briefly try to describe what it is.

When you eat, your blood sugar (glucose) level naturally rises. This in turn triggers the pancreas to secrete the hormone insulin, which stimulates your body's cells to take in and store glucose. In people who are said to be 'insulin resistant', the cells resist the hormone's efforts

> **What do you do if you've succumbed to the unthinkable, and eaten something really, really disgusting? Well, don't feel bad about it – guilt isn't going to help! If the offending morsel is still in your mouth, here's a mean little trick which may help: hold it there for at least 30 seconds. Slowly, it will taste worse and worse! But remember, with the LifePoints Diet, you can always live to fight another day, because it's a gentle process of re-education.**

to transport sugar into them from the bloodstream. Therefore, more insulin must be secreted to do the job. This situation may eventually precipitate serious health problems, including the adult form of diabetes, high blood pressure and heart disease. No one knows how many people suffer from insulin resistance. The condition is thought to be largely a result of obesity, lack of exercise, smoking and ageing, though there's also a genetic element. Weight loss and exercise can certainly lessen insulin resistance.

So much for the facts. Now for the hype! Some authors claim that eating carbohydrate-rich food stimulates insulin secretion (correct) which in turn triggers weight gain in the small proportion of the population who may be insulin resistant (by no means proven). If true – and it's a big if – food which causes blood sugar to rise at a faster rate, and to stay high for longer periods, could be more likely to provoke greater insulin secretion and therefore fat deposition. The glycaemic index measures precisely that ability in foods to raise blood sugar levels. The higher the food's glycaemic index, the greater your blood sugar levels. Here is a ranking of some common foods according to their glycaemic index – note how preparation methods can radically change the figures.

HOW THEY COMPARE – GLYCAEMIC INDEX FIGURES FOR VARIOUS FOODS

Food	Glycaemic Index (*lower is better*)
Cherries	32
Plum	34
Pearl barley	36
Grapefruit	36
Lentils	38
Butter beans	46
Chick peas	47

Food	Glycaemic Index
Milk, whole	49
Apple	52
Ice cream	52
Yogurt	52
Haricot beans	54
Orange	59
Pinto beans	60
Chick peas, canned	60
Spaghetti, whole	61
Grapes	62
Macaroni	64
Spaghetti, white	67
Yams	74
Kidney beans, canned	74
New potatoes	80
Sweet corn	80
White rice	81
Brown rice	81
Banana	84
Oatmeal porridge	89
Rolled oats	89
Raisin	93
White bread*	100

* White bread is the 'reference' food and set at 100, other foods are compared with it

Food	Glycaemic Index
Millet	103
Puffed wheat	110
Potatoes, instant	116
Corn flakes	121
Honey	126
Puffed rice	132

You may think that all this sounds rather tenuous, and indeed it is. The facts of the matter are much more murky. Does insulin resistance cause obesity – or does obesity cause insulin resistance, as many experts believe? While it's true that insulin plays an important role in fat metabolism, where is the scientific *evidence* that eating carbohydrates can cause insulin-related weight gain? So far, convincing evidence simply hasn't been presented – which is rather strange for such an allegedly revolutionary theory! In fact, many good studies have shown exactly the opposite – that switching to a high-carbohydrate, low-fat diet will indeed lead to worthwhile weight loss.

> **Everytime you fancy eating a chocolate bar, have a baked potato topped with baked beans . . . It takes longer to eat than the snack bar, has only 1 RiskPoint, compared to 35 for the snack bar, and at 20 has five times the LifePoints of the chocolate!**

So is there any use for the glycaemic index? Yes, there is. The concept was first proposed by German scientists back in 1973, when they noted that various carbohydrate foodstuffs produced different blood sugar responses in individuals.[36] Before then, all scientists had assumed that complex carbohydrates (e.g. wheat) were healthier for diabetics than simple carbohydrates (e.g. sugar). Unfortunately, this simple proposition had never actually been put to the test.[37] When it was, conventional wisdom seemed to be overturned – for example, the kind of sugar found in fruit (fructose) has a glycaemic index of 30, table sugar 86, and white bread 100. Which means that white bread is worse than fruit sugar in terms of glucose control for diabetics!

So for diabetics the glycaemic index may indeed be a useful tool for more accurately gauging the likely effect of various foods on their blood sugar level. However, even here there are some significant problems. The glycaemic index is calculated in the laboratory using human subjects, who are fed a test food and then asked to give six blood samples over two hours. The blood is analysed and the results computed to produce a number – the glycaemic index. It all sounds very neat and tidy, but in the real world things aren't so simple:

- Humans differ very considerably in their response to food – the same food can produce a four-fold variation in glycaemic response between different people[38]
- The method of preparing or cooking the food can greatly alter the food's glycaemic index.[39] In particular, the particle size of the food (e.g. if it's puréed) can make a considerable difference to the body's blood sugar response, and hence to the glycaemic index
- Even within the same food, different strains can produce very different results. For example, new potatoes have a glycaemic index of 80, but russett potatoes are 116 – nearly 50 per cent higher
- The glycaemic index is calculated by feeding people one food at a time. But outside of the laboratory people don't eat like that. For example, a fatty meal will lengthen the time food takes to pass through the upper gastrointestinal tract, and so produce a lower glycaemic response.[40] Protein, on the other hand, will increase the body's insulin secretion, leading to more rapid glucose processing.

Taking all this into account, what use is the glycaemic index for dieters? Choosing your diet exclusively on the basis of a food's glycaemic index isn't a good idea. There are currently too many uncertainties associated with it, not least of which the fact that you'd probably end up eating a diet which would be too high in fat. And only about 200 foods have so far been analysed, which gives you a very small menu to choose from!

To summarize: If the glycaemic index ever becomes a genuinely useful dieting tool, with universal practicality, you can be sure that we will incorporate it into the LifePoints system. Until then, knowing the glycaemic index of some selected foodstuffs may be useful to 'fine tune' your diet. In particular, foods with a low glycaemic index (remember – lower is better) have been shown to produce a feeling of fullness and satisfaction after consumption.[41] And given two foods with roughly equal LifePoint and RiskPoint values, it would seem judicious to prefer the one which produces the lower rise in blood sugar, i.e. the one with the lower glycaemic index. Finally, if you're concerned about the possible impact of carbohydrates on your insulin secretion – and hence on your weight control – here's some useful advice:

- Try a nibble! Changing your food consumption pattern can have a very profound effect on insulin levels. When scientists fed two groups of volunteers either three meals or 17 snacks every day, they were amazed to find that the people who snacked constantly had lowered their cholesterol by 15 per cent, and slashed their average blood insulin levels by nearly 28 per cent![42] If you choose to try this, you must ensure that you're eating *healthy* snacks – which is, of course, where the LifePoints counter can really help.

> **If you are a bread lover, transform it from a mediocre rating (most commercial breads) to a food that really scores high on LifePoints. How? Simply learn to make your own – an evening's work – and add high-Lifepoints ingredients such as beansprouts, molasses, dried fruits, wheat germ . . . even sauerkraut!**

LifePoints – Beyond the Myth of the Balanced Diet

Just a few years ago, a senior figure in Britain's Department of Health gave a talk during which the following comments were made. See if you can guess what's wrong with them!

'The public particularly mistrusts butter, milk, cheese and hard margarines and cooking fats . . . These foods have an unhealthy image. *Of course there is nothing unhealthy about any of these foods.*'

'The perjorative term [junk food] indicates how evil, bad for you and unhealthy these foods are. But are they? . . . Obvious junk foods are crisps, chips, hamburgers, sausages, meat pies, fish fried in batter, fry-ups and grills. *None of these are devoid of nutrients.*'

'Our advice must be to aim for *a balanced diet.* There are no healthy or unhealthy foods; "health" and "organic" foods have no scientific meaning.'[43]

The italics are ours, used to emphasize what are – to us – the most outrageous opinions of the official's speech. But this person wasn't a lone maverick, nor some sort of dietary reactionary. Far from it – all he was doing was voicing the official view which, from time immemorial, has held that 'there are no good foods or bad foods'. Sometimes, when we give public lectures, we quote these remarks. And we add: 'Yes, and eating Bart Simpson's shorts is fine too . . . providing they're part of *a balanced diet!*'

Plain common sense surely tells us that some foods are indeed better for us than others. When the American Dietetic Association released

> **Make the switch from milkshakes to Smoothies. A milkshake can have about 49 RiskPoints; our Melon and Apricot Smoothie page 134 has a mere 2 RiskPoints but a healthy 27 LifePoints per serving. Make your own favourites using high-LifePoints foods from the LifePoints counter.**

the results of a recent public opinion survey into attitudes towards food, they found that three out of four people surveyed did indeed believe that there are 'good' and 'bad' foods. That finding must have vexed officials everywhere, because for years they've been trying to tell us precisely the opposite – that virtually any food can be part of a 'well-balanced' diet.

Well, *someone* out there must be happily eating that mythical 'well-balanced' diet, because we hear so much about it all the time. Someone out there must be eating all the burgers, all the french fries, all the ice cream, all the high-fat products, and all the other foods we are so regularly told are just fine for us 'when eaten as part of a balanced diet'.

> **The most convenient food in the world is completely natural and – you guessed it – high in Lifepoints, low in RiskPoints. What is easier than to peel a banana, polish and crunch an apple, or munch your way leisurely through a handful of dried apricots, figs, currants or dates.**

But so far, we've never met them.

All we see is evidence of people eating bad foods, and becoming ill. Conversely, we see scientific studies following the health of people who eat good foods – and they *stay* healthy.

Think critically for a moment about the myth of the 'balanced diet', and you'll soon realize just how preposterous it is. Stripped of its officialese, it's really having us believe that 'No food can be considered to be "good" or "bad", because virtually *any* food can be consumed providing it is done in the context of a balanced diet.' Now, follow this logic with us for a moment, and you'll soon see just how daft it really is.

If any food is OK, as long as it's part of a balanced diet, then food such as burgers, fries and milkshakes are fine . . . providing they are 'balanced' by the consumption of other foods.

All right. But precisely what 'other foods'? That's never made clear. We can assume, however, that those mysterious 'other foods' contain the health-enhancing nutrients which burgers, fries and shakes singularly lack. We can also assume that those 'other foods' *don't* contain the harmful fats and other anti-nutrients which burgers, fries and shakes most certainly do contain. In other words, those 'other foods' are *good* foods!

Furthermore, junk foods such as these contain absolutely no nutrients which can't be obtained from other food sources. Indeed, there are plenty of other foods which contain the nutrients that are found in junk food – but which *don't* contain all the unhealthy fats and other anti-nutrient factors. So junk food makes no uniquely valuable contribution towards our overall good nutritional status, but it *does* contribute several undesirable anti-nutrients which we could well do without. In our book, that's a pretty accurate definition of a 'bad' food!

So stripped down to basics, what they're actually saying is: 'It's OK to eat bad foods, as long as you also eat good foods.' To which we make a one-word reply:

Balderdash!

The myth of the 'balanced diet' is really trying to persuade us to doubt our own very trustworthy instincts about food. It is trying to convince us that eating almost *any* kind of food, no matter how unwholesome, is acceptable – providing it is 'balanced' by the consumption of some magical super-healthy antidote food later on. What absolute nonsense. There is no scientific evidence that this 'magical antidote' theory of healthy eating is anything other than a rather cruel – and deceptive – fairy tale. Don't swallow it!

The bottom line is this: We don't talk about a 'balanced' diet . . . whatever that much-abused phrase actually means. Instead, we talk about a *good* diet! And how do you eat a good diet? Easy – by eating good food. And how can you tell the good food from the rest? That's easy too – for the first time ever, you have the power to start doing that – quite literally – at your fingertips . . .

ALL ABOUT LIFEPOINTS

It seems extraordinary to think that before LifePoints, there was no simple way to easily check the nutritional worth of the food you ate. Although the raw data for food composition and the computing power to attempt the task were certainly available, the biggest problem was simply the prevailing mind-set character-ized by that endlessly- repeated mantra: 'There are no good foods or bad foods, only good diets and bad diets.' Obviously, if there weren't any good foods or bad foods, there was no point in trying to rate them as such.

We thought differently. Applying decades of human population studies, we sought to assemble a picture of the major healthy and unhealthy factors in the human diet. For example, the evidence is overwhelming that people who consume significant quantities of saturated fat have a high incidence of heart disease – so saturated fat is clearly a major risk factor in our diets. On the other hand, people who eat foods that are high in the antioxidant beta-carotene (see page 53) have much less heart disease and fewer cancers – which indicates that beta-carotene is one of the important health protectors. Many of these nutritional factors will already be familiar to you. However, *never before* have you had the opportunity to see how they all add up to make a healthy or unhealthy food. Now, you can.

> **On Sunday evening, make-up the recipe for Fruit and Cereal Snack Bars (page 127), slice into six servings and wrap each one individually. Every morning, place one in your handbag or briefcase and eat it instead of the snack bar you might otherwise buy.**

The task of producing Life-Point numbers for each of the foods in this book began with a major computational effort. Over the course of several months, computers performed countless millions of calculations, and gradually the raw data began to take shape. For the first time, we began to see patterns emerging – and surprises too. Food that we had always believed to be 'healthy' sometimes proved to be anything but. And frequently, we found ourselves bestowing a new, healthy respect on modest foodstuffs which we'd hitherto overlooked. We're certain you will share these experiences as you become familiar with the LifePoints system. Indeed, we hope you share the thrill we first felt when you realize just how effective and uncomplicated it is to use.

What do LifePoints actually measure? People sometimes expect the system to be measured in calories or some other familiar unit, and are puzzled when it isn't. Well, think about it like this. Instead of measuring just one nutrient, LifePoints

> **Popcorn can be the wholegrain snack it was meant to be if you air-pop it rather than oil-pop it. Instead of being a vehicle for butter, it can be seasoned with sweet spices, paprika, nutritional yeast flakes or soy sauce.**

measures *lots* of them. First, we calculate an overall nutritional profile for the food being analysed, in its most common serving size. Next, we use a proprietary computer algorithm to compare the nutritional profile of that food with its respective 'ideal' nutritional profile, and see how it fits. A good fit earns lots of LifePoints – a bad one earns none. It is important to emphasize that we're not just adding up all the nutrients in the food. That would produce a misleading result, since foods which contain very large amounts of just one or two nutrients would come out far too favourably. A food which has a high LifePoints number provides you with *lots* of nutrients in *beneficial* amounts. And if that food is also low in RiskPoints, then it's a *good* food. Simple, isn't it? These two numbers – LifePoints and RiskPoints – instantly provide you with a dynamic and enlightening picture of any food you care to look up! Now let's briefly describe the importance of the nutrients included in the LifePoints ratings system.

● **Beta-carotene** The plant form of vitamin A, it functions as a powerful antioxidant and free radical quencher in the human body. The evidence is overwhelming that beta-carotene is one of the most important nutritional factors in your armoury against ill-health. Popularly, beta-carotene is sometimes known as a 'cancer killer'. Men who eat very little beta-carotene have been shown to be seven times more likely to contract lung cancer than men whose diets are rich in it. In women, beta-carotene seems to be able to thwart cervical cancer. Further, epidemiological evidence indicates that it can also reduce the incidence of cancers of the larynx, bladder, oesophagus, stomach, colorectum and prostate gland.

Today, we hear a great deal about antioxidants and free radicals. In recent years scientists have begun to appreciate just how crucial antioxidants are to our health. The LifePoints Diet delivers you a diet which is *naturally* high in many of the most powerful antioxidants. First, let's describe what they are.

In the popular media, free radicals are often characterized as 'bad', but as in so many things, this is only partly true. The 'free radical theory' was first proposed as long ago as 1954 by Dr Denham Harman, latterly professor of medicine and biochemistry at the University of Nebraska. He discovered that radiation caused accelerated ageing, and also created an excess of free radicals in body cells. What is a free radical? Simply, an atom or molecule with an unpaired electron. It is inherently unstable, as it continually searches for another molecule to which to attach itself. Gerontologist Alex Comfort wittily compared a free radical to a convention delegate away from his wife: 'a highly reactive chemical agent that will combine with anything that's around'. Free radicals trigger a chain reaction that 'rusts' the body. Free radicals can damage cell membranes, proteins, carbohydrates, and deoxyribonucleic acid (DNA) – the genetic material of the cell and of life itself. Up to now, some 60 diseases have been associated with free radical activity, including Alzheimer's, heart disease, arthritis, multiple sclerosis and eye cataracts. Even 'liver spots – areas of brown skin which appear on your hands and arms later in life – are connected to free radical activity. Although the body naturally produces free radicals, other substances, such as cigarette smoke, radiation, air pollution, herbicides, artificial flavorings, chlorine, rancid fats, alcohol and toxic heavy metals are also causes of free radical formation.

> **Too rushed for breakfast? Your blood sugar levels will really go wild about mid-morning. Why not pack a breakfast that you can eat as soon as you get to work instead of buying junk to eat on the train.**

Free radicals aren't all bad, however. There is persuasive evidence that the basic chemicals of life first originated in the 'primeval soup' from a series of free radical reactions, triggered by ionizing radiation from the sun. This would explain why free radical reactions are so pervasive in nature. They enable genetic mutations to occur, and so play a pivotal role in the process of evolution. And your body *deliberately* produces free radicals when it wants to kill invading organisms, as part of its immune and inflammatory responses. Obviously your body needs a system to manage free radicals effectively and, in particular, there has to be an effective protective and scavenging system to ensure that they don't get out of control. And that's what antioxidants do.

Ageing isn't simply about crow's feet and turkey jowls. The ageing process brings about many serious changes in the human body. In fact, after the age of 28, the greatest single risk factor for disease and death is the ageing process itself.[44] It is shocking to realize that, if one day all the major causes of premature death were eliminated, the average human lifespan would *still* be only 85 years.[45] And the only way we're going to extend that is by tackling the ageing process itself.

The process of human ageing isn't fully understood, by any means. But there's no doubt that one very important aspect of the ageing process is the damage that free radicals inflict on the human body. When things get out of balance between free radicals (pro-oxidants) and antioxidants, problems begin. If you're low on antioxidants, then you're wide open to free radical attack. In fact, many scientists now suspect that what we call 'ageing' is simply the final result of many free radical reactions going on continuously through our cells and tissues.[46] If that view is correct, then the ageing process might be amenable to alleviation, and what we today consider to be an inevitable process, might tomorrow be considered a *disease* process – and treated accordingly.

Several scientific studies have already shown that dietary antioxidants can increase lifespan.[47] There's also powerful evidence from human populations that those people who take in bountiful amounts of natural antioxidants suffer far less from many killers, such as cancer and heart disease. In America, the Alliance for Ageing Research (which is a non-profit public health organization) recently assembled a panel of leading medical researchers, nutritionists and consumer safety experts to examine antioxidants and ageing. They reviewed over 200 clinical and epidemiologic studies conducted over the past two decades, and concluded that 'A diet rich in antioxidants, including beta-carotene and vitamins C and E, is effective in guarding against heart disease, cancer, cataracts and other conditions associated with ageing.[48] The LifePoints Diet provides you with a diet that is naturally high in these major antioxidants.

STAYING YOUNGER, LONGER – OUR SIX GOLDEN RULES	
1	Eat a diet high in natural antioxidants – at least 100 LifePoints a day.
2	Go for quality, not quantity – your food must be fresh and wholesome, organic if possible.
3	Use it or lose it! Stretch both your body and your mind daily.
4	Think young! Keep your aspirations alive and nurture your ambitions – every day you get better and better!
5	Never retire! But a change is as good as a rest, so change careers every six years.
6	Variety is the spice of your (sex) life – remember romance isn't just for teenagers!

Beta-carotene is one such powerful natural antioxidant. Found in plants, it is turned into vitamin A in the wall of the small intestine during digestion. Of the several hundred naturally occurring carotenoids, the most widespread and most active form is beta-carotene. Foods which contain beta-carotene can be consumed in plentiful amounts without fear of toxicity. Beta-carotene is also:

- Essential for good eyesight
- Vital for tissue growth and bone development
- Used to maintain the integrity of mucous membranes, thus building a barrier against infection
- Necessary for the proper growth and functioning of the reproductive system.

Taking beta-carotene, and indeed all nutrients, in their natural form is very important. In nature, *nothing works in isolation*. This was dramatically underlined recently when the results of a long-awaited major study came to the startling conclusion that high doses of beta-carotene, when taken in capsule form, may actually *raise* the risk of cancer rather than lower it. The first indication that a foodstuff may possess health-promoting properties frequently comes from epidemiological studies on human populations. Scientists usually react to this sort of information by trying to isolate the exact chemical or substance in the food which confers this benefit. At the end of the process is, all too often, the quest for yet another pill. As the news wires put it: 'Hopes are high that researchers may someday find dread cancers could be avoided simply by taking a daily pill . . .'[49]

But strange and unexpected things happen when you extract one nutrient in isolation. The most recent study was intended to show whether beta-carotene protects smokers from lung cancer. Instead, it found that those taking the isolated vitamin *increased* their lung cancer risk by 18 per cent. The 10-year, $43-million study was conducted on 29,133 male cigarette smokers who lived in Finland. Smokers were chosen because they are already at high risk of lung cancer, and beta-carotene appeared to be especially promising as a way to lower the chance of this disease. At this stage, no one can say for sure why the researchers found this effect. But don't let's misunderstand this. This single study does *not* suggest that foods which naturally supply a plentiful amount of beta-carotene may increase your risk of cancer. Quite the opposite. Decades of studies tracking the health of thousands of people prove the wisdom of eating beta-carotene-rich foods. But whether it's wise to replace this sort of food with a pill . . . well, that's anyone's guess. What we can repeat, however, is that no nutrient works in isolation in nature. The LifePoints system gives you a way of assessing the broad nutritional profile of many different kinds of food. It's a wholistic approach – and the healthiest.

• **Vitamin C**   Long considered as only relevant to the prevention of scurvy, there is now abundant evidence that a first-class intake of vitamin C can help to prevent a wide range of human diseases. Humans are one of the few species unable to synthesize vitamin C internally, and therefore we need to be certain of a regular, high-quality dietary intake. Vitamin C is also a very effective antioxidant and free radical quencher. You can even see it at work for yourself. Cut an apple in half, and put one half aside. Pour lemon juice, which is high in vitamin C, on the other half.

The half without the lemon juice will go brown through oxidation much faster than the half which is protected by the antioxidant vitamin C. In a recent study conducted at the University of California at Berkeley, scientists isolated plasma from human blood, incubated it at body temperature and added a chemical that is known to produce free radicals as it decomposes. When vitamin C was added it neutralized 100 per cent of the free radicals generated. Vitamin C also:

- Assists in the production of collagen, a protein which is the body's building block for all connective tissue, cartilage, bones, teeth, skin and tendons
- Helps wounds, fractures, bruises and haemorrhages heal
- Maintains function of the immune system
- Greatly facilitates the absorption of iron from the diet
- Assists haemoglobin and red blood cell production
- Is an essential co-factor for metabolism of many other nutrients
- Helps the body cope with physiological and psychological stress.

Further, vitamin C seems to block the formation of nitrosamines. Nitrates and nitrites are added to foods to give colour, flavour and to act as preservatives (E249–E252). During digestion these substances are converted by the human body into nitrosamines, which are known to be powerful cancer-causing chemicals (they are particularly associated with cancers of the stomach and oesophagus). The good news is that if a vitamin C-rich food is taken at the same time as foods containing nitrates or nitrites, then the production of nitrosamines is greatly reduced. It has also been found that women with abnormal cervical smear results often have low amounts of vitamin C in their body. This may shed new light on the underlying damage caused by smoking, because it has long been established that women who smoke have higher levels of cervical cancer. Smoking impairs the absorption of vitamin C but also requires that you take in more vitamin C to minimize the effects of it as a pollutant.

● **Thiamin** Also called thiamine or vitamin B1, thiamin was discovered to be the nutritional factor responsible for preventing the disease beriberi (Singhalese for 'I cannot', meaning that the sufferer is too ill to do anything). Epidemics of beriberi were produced in Asia by eating a diet of white polished rice, where all the nutritional content of the outer layers of rice is discarded during processing. Although beriberi is primarily a disease of tropical countries, nutritional deficiencies of thiamin are also seen in the West – especially amongst people who eat a typically highly refined, junk food diet. In the body, thiamin functions to:

- Convert carbohydrate into energy for the muscles and nervous system
- Keep mucous membranes healthy
- Maintain a positive mental state and may assist learning capacity.

● **Riboflavin** Also known as vitamin B2, riboflavin was first observed in 1879 as a greenish fluorescent pigment present in milk, but its function was not fully understood until 1932. It is often found in combination with other B-group vitamins and, since it is not stored in the human body for any period of time, it is vital that your diet supplies regular amounts. A deficiency will result in cracked and scaly skin; soreness of lips, mouth and tongue; and sometimes heightened sensitivity to light, watering of eyes, or conjunctivitis. In the body, riboflavin works:

- With other vitamins and enzymes in the utilization of energy from food
- To keep mucous membranes healthy
- As a key component in normal tissue respiration.

● **Niacin** Also called vitamin B3, niacin is the collective name for nicotinamide (niacinamide) and nicotinic acid. Its importance was realized in 1937 when it was discovered that the disease pellagra was caused by niacin deficiency. Lack of niacin in the diet can also lead to fatigue and muscle weakness, loss of appetite and mental unbalance. In the body it plays an important role in:

- The release of energy from carbohydrates, fats and proteins
- DNA synthesis

- Keeping the skin, nerves and digestive systems working healthily.

● **Vitamin B6** Also known as pyridoxine, vitamin B6 is (in common with other B-group vitamins) soluble in water. This means that the body's storage capacity for B6 is limited, and we need to ensure a good daily dietary intake. It works in the body to:

- Manufacture and convert amino acids and metabolize protein
- Produce haemoglobin
- Convert the amino acid tryptophan to niacin
- Facilitate the release of glycogen for energy from the liver and muscles
- Help the body process linoleic acid (an essential fatty acid)
- Help build and maintain the integrity of the nervous system and brain.

● **Vitamin B12** Also called cobalamin, this vitamin is manufactured by micro-organisms such as yeasts, bacteria, moulds and some algae. The human body can store this vitamin for considerable periods (five to six years) so a daily dietary source is therefore not essential. In addition, the healthy body recycles this vitamin very effectively, recovering it from bile and other intestinal secretions, which is why the dietary requirement is so low (being measured in millionths of a gram). However, B12 deficiency is an occasional problem for people on restricted diets, and in view of its importance, it is wise to consume a known B12 food source from time to time. Its functions in the body are to:

- Facilitate the normal metabolic function of all cells
- Work with folate (see below) to prevent anaemia
- Assist in the process of DNA synthesis
- Promote the growth and normal functioning of the nervous system.

● **Folate** Folate and folacin (sometimes called vitamin B9) are the names used to describe a group of substances which are chemically similar to folic acid. Its importance to growth and the prevention of anaemia was established in 1946. The name 'folate' comes from the latin word *folium*, meaning a leaf, which should tell us something about the best sources of this vitamin. In the body, it:

- Plays an essential role in the formation of DNA and RNA, the two chemical substances involved in the genetic transmission of characteristics from parent to child.
- Functions together with vitamin B12 in amino acid synthesis
- Is essential for the formation of red and white blood cells
- Contributes to the formation of haem, the iron constituent of haemoglobin.

● **Calcium**   The most plentiful mineral in the human body, calcium amounts to one kilogram or so of the average adult's weight. Ninety-nine per cent is deposited in the bones and teeth, with the remainder fulfilling essential regulatory functions in the blood and cellular fluids. The body stores its skeletal calcium in two ways: in the non-exchangeable pool (calcium which is on 'long-term deposit' in the bones) and in the exchangeable pool – which can act as a short-term buffer to smooth over the peaks and troughs in the day-to-day dietary calcium intakes. If dietary intake is consistently too low then the exchangeable pool of calcium will become so depleted that the calcium on 'long-term deposit' in the bones will be put to use, thus inducing bone degeneration.

Although calcium is often thought of as the 'bone mineral', the 1 per cent of serum calcium in the human body (calcium held outside the skeletal structure) is responsible for a vital and complex range of tasks. Calcium is clearly a critical nutrient, and we all need to ensure that we have an intake. Many people erroneously believe that the consumption of heroic quantities of dairy produce is the only way to prevent bone-depleting afflictions such as osteoporosis. This is not so – the landmark China Study we've already mentioned (see page 39) showed that although the Chinese take in only half the amount of calcium that Westerners do, osteoporosis is rare in China. Why should this be? Well, most Chinese eat no dairy products and instead get all their calcium from vegetables. This is why we've included the calcium content of all foods in the LifePoints equation. We'd like you to get a good calcium intake from a wide variety of foods, rather than assuming that large amounts of milk and dairy products will protect you. In fact, studies among Western vegetarians and meat-eaters show that people who eat meat and dairy products are significantly more at risk of bone loss than non-meat eaters. Calcium also functions in the body to:

- Help build and maintain bones and teeth
- Help control transport of chemicals across cell membranes
- Facilitate the release of neurotransmitters at synapses
- Influence the function of protein hormones and enzymes
- Help regulate heartbeat and muscle tone
- Initiate blood clotting.

● **Iron** We all know that iron prevents anaemia and is essential for haemoglobin production. As such, it is involved in the transportation of oxygen from the lungs to the body's tissues, it transports and stores oxygen in the muscles, and is involved in the proper functioning of the immune system and intellect. Iron deficiency is the most common of all deficiency diseases in both developing and developed countries. Scientists vary in their estimate of what precisely constitutes a state of 'iron depletion', but the general cut-off point is variously calculated to lie between 12 and 25 micrograms of ferritin (one of the chief iron storage forms) per litre of plasma. In Britain, a recent survey showed that 34 per cent of all women had a ferritin level which was under 25mcg/l, and 16 per cent had less than 13mcg/l. Amongst men, only 6 per cent had a value of less than 25mcg/l, and 3 per cent less than 13mcg/l.

These figures reflect the fact that iron is well conserved by the body (90 per cent of the 3 to 5 grams in our bodies is continually recycled). The major cause of iron depletion is loss of blood itself – as in menstruation, which on average causes about half a milligram of iron to be lost for every day of the period. However, this can vary very widely (losses as high as 1.4 milligrams a day have been reported) so the official recommended daily allowances for women attempt to take this into account by building in a generous 'safety margin'. For example, an iron intake of 10.8 milligrams a day appears to meet the needs of 86 per cent of all menstruating women[50] yet the official American recommended daily allowance has been set at 15 milligrams a day in an attempt to meet the needs of the remaining 14 per cent. This is, in fact, an uneasy compromise because even at this level of iron consumption, 5 per cent of women who have very heavy periods will not have an adequate intake to replace losses. At this point, the officials either suggest that women with higher blood losses appear to compensate with an increased rate of iron absorption from their diets (American) or 'the most practical way of meeting their high iron requirements would be to take iron supplements' (British). This illustrates well the dilemma facing officials whose task it is to set uniform nutritional intakes for a population whose individual needs naturally vary very widely indeed.

The rate of absorption of iron from the diet can be significantly affected, for better or worse, by several factors:

- First, the rate of iron absorption is controlled by the degree to which iron is actually *needed* by the body. Normally, only 5 to 15 per cent of the iron in food is actually absorbed; but this can rise to 50 per cent in cases of iron deficiency.
- Foods containing vitamin C will considerably increase iron absorption. Iron must be delivered in a soluble form to the small intestine if it is to be absorbed, and vitamin C can make sure that non-haem iron (the sort found in plant foods) remains soluble in the acidic environment normally found there. Other organic acids found in fruit and vegetables, such as malic acid and citric acid, are also thought to possess this iron-enhancing attribute. The effect is substantial: adding 60 milligrams of vitamin C to a meal of rice has been shown to more than triple the absorption of iron; adding the same amount to a meal of corn enhances absorption fivefold. The LifePoints formula includes both iron and vitamin C.
- The tannin in tea can significantly reduce the absorption of iron, by combining with it to form insoluble iron compounds. The food preservative EDTA can also exercise the same inhibitory effect. Both of these factors can reduce assimilation by as much as 50 per cent.

- **Zinc** The human body contains a mere 2 grams of zinc, distributed in the tissues in varying concentrations. Its importance to good human nutrition has only been recognized in recent years (the first reports appeared in 1963). Low zinc status often manifests in a decrease in the senses of taste and smell, wounds take longer to heal, and children fail to grow properly. This is because, in the human body, zinc is:

- An essential component of many enzymes which work with red blood cells to transport carbon dioxide from tissues to lungs
- A vital factor in many key life processes, such as our immune function and the expression of genetic information.

In addition to all the nutrients mentioned above, the LifePoints number also assesses foods for their fibre content (which, as you must know, imparts a whole host of health benefits, ranging from the prevention of various forms of cancer, to lowering blood cholesterol and preventing constipation) and their protein content. *A high LifePoints number indicates that the food concerned is a beneficial source of nutrients. A low number indicates that it is a poor source.*

Now you know the basics of the LifePoints food control system. The next thing is to get it working for you!

PART TWO: THE LIFEPOINTS KICK-START

The moment has arrived! It's time to put the past behind you and discover a healthy new way of eating – and living. On this voyage of discovery, the LifePoints system will be your friend and guide.

Because people are so accustomed to diets which boss them around and tell them precisely what they may or may not eat, they sometimes find the freedom of the LifePoints system rather strange. To help you adjust to life outside 'diet prison', we've created the LifePoints Kick-Start, which gently holds your hand as we walk through the first seven days of your diet, and then gives you some good ideas for the future (for example, how to adapt your favourite recipes to make them high LifePoints recipes). First, let's make the principles of the LifePoints Diet absolutely clear.

All the foods in the listings in Part Five have been carefully analysed to reveal their nutritional profile. Each food has two numbers:

- **The LifePoints number is a measure of the food's healthy components – the higher the number, the healthier the food.**
- **The RiskPoints number is a measure of the food's unhealthy components – the higher the number, the more unhealthy the food.**

So a food with high RiskPoints and no LifePoints is a 'bad' food. Similarly, a food with high LifePoints and no RiskPoints is a 'good' food. Your aim is to maximize the number of LifePoints you consume, while not exceeding the RiskPoints limit. How many RiskPoints and LifePoints should you consume? It's simple . . .

Your LifePoints target should be at least 100 per day

Your initial RiskPoints limit should be 75 per day while you're dieting, and to suit thereafter

---

That's all the adding up you have to do! Now you know the way the LifePoints system works. It's much easier than calorie-counting, because you don't have to add up to 1000 or more. And, uniquely, the LifePoints system gives you a feeling for the food itself. Use it for just a day or two, and you'll find that your own instincts for good food and bad food are revived and developed. That's why we say LifePoints is an empowering system. Now let's lay down a few ground rules:

THE THREE LIFEPOINTS LAWS

1 *Eat healthily!* Dieters are notoriously unhealthy eaters. Skipping breakfast and lunch, then gorging on a mid-afternoon chocolate bar is **not** healthy – and is not slimming either. Your first and prime objective is to score at least 100 LifePoints – more if you can. In the first week you'll see that every day scores at least 200 LifePoints . . . so it's not hard!

2 *Eat for variety!* For your convenience we have divided foods into six major groups. To eat a healthy and varied diet, you *must* choose foods from the first four groups. Groups 5 and 6 are optional. The suggested number of servings per day from each group is listed below:

Group 1	Fruit and Fruit Juices	3 servings
Group 2	Cereals, Grains and Pasta	4 servings
Group 3	Vegetables and Vegetable Products	4 servings
Group 4	Legumes, Nuts and Seeds	3 servings
Group 5	Meat, Fish and Dairy	optional
Group 6	Drinks, Desserts, Snacks and Sauces	optional

3 *Don't be boring!* We'll say it again – variety is the keynote of healthy eating. To encourage you to eat as wide a variety as possible, you must observe this rule: the LifePoints for any foodstuff can only be counted once, no matter how often you eat that food during the day. This means that if you eat the same food twice, only its RiskPoints count for the second helping. In other words, don't try to cheat the system by eating 10 servings of broccoli for 120 LifePoints and only 10 RiskPoints! (If you ever did eat ten helpings of broccoli, using this simple rule you'd accumulate 10 RiskPoints but only 12 LifePoints.) Foods are listed in common serving sizes, but it's quite acceptable to halve or even quarter the servings, providing you similarly reduce the associated RiskPoints and LifePoints.

SUPERCHARGING THE SYSTEM

The LifePoints system is very flexible, and can be customized to suit your individual requirements. Here we give some advice on personalizing LifePoints to suit you, and answer some common questions.

How does weight loss occur?

In several natural ways. First, you'll be eating a broad and varied diet which is low in fat – probably much lower than you're used to. The amount, and type, of fat you consume is controlled by the RiskPoints number. Since everyone is different – a fact that most other diets don't seem to recognize – we suggest you start at a RiskPoints limit of 75 per day during weight loss, but this limit can be adjusted to suit your individual requirements, using the table below as a guide. People respond very individually to diet therapy, so a little experimentation and fine tuning might be necessary. Obviously, you should also seek the advice of your medical or health specialist when formulating an effective therapy.

A total of 75 RiskPoints will provide no more than 30 grams of fat in your diet (which is about 12 per cent of your calorie intake for someone taking in 2200 calories a day). At other times, a RiskPoints limit of 100 will ensure that your diet is still healthily low in fat, and weight loss will probably continue. Note that the RiskPoints number doesn't *just* measure the total amount of fat you consume – it also steers you away from food which is unhealthily high in saturated fat. If you veer that way, you'll quickly find that you're over your limit!

Your RiskPoints Limit	Potential For Weight Loss
75	Allows 30 grams of fat a day – the lowest suggested limit
100	Allows 40 grams of fat a day – maintains weight loss
125	Allows 50 grams of fat a day – gradual weight loss still occurs[51]

In addition to this, when you eat complex carbohydrates – which tend to be found in food which is high in LifePoints – you're naturally reducing your calorie intake, without having to perform all those mental gymnastics. Carbohydrate-rich meals are naturally low in calories. As you may know, carbohydrates yield only 4 calories per gram, but fat provides twice as many with 9 calories. So gram for gram, or ounce for ounce, carbohydrate-rich food is naturally a better deal for the slimmer.

The LifePoints Diet also helps you lose weight in another important way. By eating complex carbohydrates, you'll do something rather magical to your body's metabolic system. Here's how nutrition expert Dr Neal Barnard explains it:

Carbohydrate-rich meals are not just low in calories. They actually change your body. They readjust your hormones, which in turn boost your metabolism and speed the burning of calories. One of these hormones is thyroid hormone. Below your Adam's apple, your thyroid gland manufactures a hormone called T4, so named because it has four iodine atoms attached. This hormone has two possible fates: it can be converted into the active form of thyroid hormone called T3, which boosts your metabolism and keeps your body burning calories, or it can be converted to an inactive hormone, called *reverse* T3. When your diet is rich in carbohydrates, more of the T4 is converted to T3, and your metabolism gets a good boost. If your diet is low in carbohydrate, more of the T4 is turned into reverse T3, resulting in a slowed metabolism. The same thing occurs during periods of very low calorie dieting or starvation. Less of the T4 is converted to T3 and more to the useless reverse T3. This is presumably the body's way of guarding its reserves of fat; when not much food is coming in, the body conserves fat and turns down production of the fat-burning hormone, T3. But a diet generous in carbohydrates keeps T3 levels high and keeps the fat fires burning.[52]

Sounds good, doesn't it? But there's more! Have you ever wondered why smokers are often so thin? Perhaps you've even harboured resentful hankerings about their gaunt physiques, and thought about taking up the weed just to trim down a bit? Well, now you can *look* like a slender smoker, without that hacking cough! As carbohydrate-rich food gradually releases sugars into the body, this stimulates the production of a neurohormone called noradrenalin, which plays an important role in instructing your body's brown fat cells (also known as brown adipose tissue) to consume stored fat. The basic function of brown fat cells is to warm the blood and distribute heat through your body, and they do this by burning fat – good news for slimmers! Scientists estimate that – when stimulated – brown fat can burn up between 200 to 400 calories a day, which would equate to a useful weight loss of about 2 pounds a month.[53] Now, smokers stimulate their brown fat cells by releasing noradrenalin into their systems. The good news is that researchers have found that the glucose released by carbohydrate-rich foods can raise your noradrenalin level by about the same amount as cigarettes![54] So next time you may be tempted to reach for a coffin-nail, reach for a carrot instead!

We're not finished yet. High-LifePoints foods serve another vital function – they tell you when to stop eating. Your body actually adjusts your appetite based on the carbohydrate content of the meals you eat. You can prove this experiment for yourself right now. First, imagine yourself with 10 chips on a plate in front of you. Eat them! Now, do you still feel hungry? Of course you do. Actually, you've just mentally consumed about 12 grams of fat – a significant amount. Let's do the experiment again, but this time imagine a large baked potato. Eat it all up, and ask yourself if you've still got room for more. Almost certainly not. Both foods had the same calorie yield. But the baked potato contained a mere 0.2 grams of fat – 60 times less than the chips! If fat made you feel full, the chips would have done so. In fact, the carbohydrate-rich potato did the trick. And so will high-LifePoints food.

How long should I try it for?

A two-week trial should be enough time for you to feel comfortable with the LifePoints Diet and to start to feel an appreciable benefit.

How much weight will I lose?

Of course, this depends mostly on you. Most diet books make rather outrageous claims about their potential for weight loss, and most of them fail to back up those claims with independent scientific evidence. The authors usually insist that their particular diet has saved their life, their hips, their bust, their marriage, their best friend's budgerigar, or something equally suspicious which you basically just have to take on trust.

As a pleasant change from all that, we'd like to mention some recent research which was independent, scientific, and may prove somewhat encouraging. In 1991, the results of the world's longest controlled human-feeding study ever to be undertaken were published.[55] Scientifically speaking, it was a beautifully designed study.[56] Thirteen women aged between 22 and 56 were randomly put into one of two groups. The first ate a low-fat diet (at about the 125 RiskPoints limit) while the second group ate a control diet (moderately calorie-restricted but not low in fat). Both groups ate the same type of food, but the low-fat group ate reduced-fat versions (e.g. low-fat yogurt instead of regular). Significantly, although the low-fat group could eat as much food as they wanted to, they actually chose to consume about 250 fewer calories a day. After 11 weeks, the subjects were given a complete break for seven weeks (a so-called 'washout' period) and then the tables were turned – the low-fat group went onto the control diet, and the former control group ate low-fat. This sort of study is called a 'crossover' study and is a powerful way of eliminating bias and individual idiosyncrasies.

The results were very encouraging. When the women went on the low-fat diet they lost twice as much weight as those on the calorie-controlled diet – about half a pound a week, 2½ kilograms in 11 weeks.

Now, of course *your* mileage may vary. This degree of weight loss may not be the fastest in the world, but it's pretty close to painless – and there's good evidence to believe that it *lasts*. As the scientists wrote:

> There is a great deal of evidence that conscious reduction in the amount of food consumed results in rapid losses of body weight; but almost invariably this lost weight is regained. Reductions in the fat content of the diet with no limitation on the amount of food consumed may lead to a more permanent weight loss than can be achieved through [conventional] dieting.

Finally, we want to add one last point about the way weight loss may occur on the LifePoints Diet. We strongly suspect that much of today's over-eating is caused not by gluttony, but simply by the body's natural quest for a highly nutritious diet. We cannot quote any scientific reference to support this hunch. Nevertheless, we believe it may be true. Wouldn't it be ironic if, in the quest for optimum nutrition, our bodies' instincts are actually precipitating one of today's major threats to our health? Of course, the LifePoints system can help here, too, by guiding us to the most nutritious foods.

What about alcohol?

Sorry, but alcohol is completely out while you're doing the LifePoints Diet. At other times, we suggest you restrict your consumption to no more than two glasses of red wine a day. In most countries, high dietary intakes of saturated fats are strongly associated with high coronary heart disease death rates. Some regions of France, however, appear to be an exception to this rule; they have low heart disease death rates despite high-fat diets. This paradox may be due to the antioxidant phenolic compounds which red wine contains (and, as we all know, the French *do* drink red wine). No other alcohol has this effect.

While losing weight, however, alcohol is not on the menu. Not only does it supply you with calories without any nutritional value ('empty calories'), it can also alter your body chemistry so as to reduce temporarily your natural ability to burn off fat.[57]

What about 'double zero' foods?

Look at the listings of foods in Part Five, and you'll see some of them have no LifePoints and no RiskPoints – double zero foods. Don't make the mistake of thinking that they can be eaten abundantly. People who are used to counting calories occasionally confuse the LifePoints system with their previous dietary regime. It's not the same at all! Double zero foods are empty foods, and have little place in your diet strategy. Remember, you have two objectives: 1) to achieve a high LifePoints score; and 2) to keep your RiskPoints within the designated limit. Double zero foods do *not* help you to achieve your primary dietary goal of a healthy LifePoints score. In fact, they're counter-productive, because they make it less likely that you'll have the appetite to eat higher-scoring foods during the day. The LifePoints system helps you *prioritize* your food intake. Double zero foods are very low priority.

Is there any need to take food supplements?

Well, we do, because we feel that even if you are eating a high-LifePoints diet, it's still important to have 'nutritional insurance'. Also, certain groups of the population have enhanced nutritional needs. In today's society, where food is so plentiful, it may seem strange to think that under-nutrition can occur at all, but the evidence shows that it can. Although you can substantially increase your overall nutrient intake by following the LifePoints system, you should still be aware that some nutrients are not particularly easy to obtain from day-to-day food sources. In particular:

- *Calcium*: if your dietary intake of this vital mineral is consistently too low then bone degeneration may occur. Many people incorrectly suppose that the consumption of copious amounts of dairy produce is the only way to prevent bone-depleting afflictions such as osteoporosis. This isn't true – strangely enough, people who eat meat and dairy products are more at risk of bone loss than non-meat eaters. Good plant food sources of calcium include blackstrap molasses, sesame seeds, tofu, green leafy vegetables such as collards, cabbage, almonds, and carob flour. Calcium is best absorbed when you have adequate vitamin D in your body (sunlight is a good source) and when there's plenty of boron in the diet (available in apples and other fresh fruits and vegetables).

- *Iron*: well conserved by the body (90 per cent of the 3 to 5 grams in our bodies is continually recycled) the major cause of iron depletion is loss of blood itself – as in menstruation. Women of childbearing years should therefore take care to eat good dietary sources, which include blackstrap molasses, pumpkin and squash seeds, spirulina, many fortified breakfast cereals; quinoa, dried mixed fruit, wheat germ, and kidney beans. Foods which contain vitamin C (e.g. fresh fruit and vegetables) will considerably increase your absorption. Several factors can significantly reduce the absorption of iron, among them tea (the tannin forms insoluble iron compounds) and the food preservative EDTA. Both of these can reduce assimilation by as much as 50 per cent.

- *Vitamin B12*: If you are eating a diet composed exclusively of plant-based foods (i.e. from the first four groups only) then make sure you sometimes consume a good source of vitamin B12, such as fortified breakfast cereal, fortified soya milk, yeast extract or fermented food such as tempeh.

Do I have to make allowances for the freshness of food?

Yes, you do. The level of nutrition you receive from your diet depends not only on what food you choose to eat, but also on how you store and cook it. This provides at least three opportunities for nutrient loss. If you lead a hectic, demanding life, you require these nutrients even more and therefore need to know how you can safeguard them. So, please, read and take to heart this advice:

- The more a foodstuff is processed, the greater the loss of natural nutrients. So buy only unprocessed wholefoods.
- If possible buy organic food, preferably from local producers. Organic foods are more likely to have their nutrients intact and, if they are from local producers, they will not have been in long storage during transit. Nutrients decay with time – so eat close to the soil! Also, the risk of pesticide residue is remote. Pesticides are poisons – their basic purpose is to kill. In an ideal world, pesticides are not supposed to leave any residue on food by the time it's ready for us to eat. But

considerable evidence indicates that the food we eat *can* be tainted with pesticide residue, even if it's been washed many times. Herbicides are often absorbed directly into the system of the plant itself, so that it is impossible to get rid of them simply by washing. Thankfully, many supermarket chains have now started to stock organic produce.

So what is organic food? The Soil Association states:

Organic food is produced responsibly, taking account of the needs of consumers, farm animals and the environment. Organic farmers produce food which:

- Is grown without artificial pesticides and fertilizers
- Tastes good rather than just looks good
- Is never irradiated
- Contains no artificial hormones, genetically manipulated organisms or unnecessary medication
- Is not over-processed to remove the goodness
- Does not contain flavourings, dyes and other additives
- Is nutritious, living food which promotes positive health and well-being.

Organic food is also better for the environment. Intensive agriculture is responsible for about 50 per cent of all water pollution (such as high nitrate levels). It has been clearly established that modern biological-organic farming methods lead both to lower leaching of nitrates into the water supply, and to lower nitrate content in vegetables.

If you can't afford to eat organic food all the time (and it *can* be very expensive), at least try to make sure that your children eat as organically as possible. Children are much more vulnerable than adults to the toxic effects of chemical residue. (NB we mention this, in passing, because we're parents ourselves – the LifePoints Diet is not intended for children.)

Here are some more tips to maximize the nutritional bang in your food:

- Do check the use-by date. Old produce will have suffered severe nutritional decay. Shopkeepers always put older stock at the front of the display – so disarrange their display, and buy from the back.

- Canning and bottling reduces the levels of vitamin C, thiamin and folic acid. Vitamin C loss continues during storage. If you have to buy canned food, do not keep it overlong. Although it may be safe to eat, its nutrients may be severely depleted.

- Avoid foods which contain sulphur dioxide as a preservative – they will have almost entirely lost their thiamin (vitamin B1) content.

- Freeze-dried foods are relatively good since there is no heating to deplete nutrients.

- Frozen foods suffer some thiamin and vitamin C loss. However the loss is less than in fresh food which has been kept for a number of days. If shopping for fresh food is a problem for you, frozen foods are probably the next best alternative, but be extra careful not to over cook them (see below).

- Choose unrefined monounsaturated oils – preferably olive oil – for cooking. Pure, refined polyunsaturated oils turn rancid more easily.

- Don't buy tinned goods which are damaged – no matter how good a bargain they appear to be. Small cracks in the lining inside the cans affect the contents, which will in turn certainly affect the delicate vitamins and other nutrients and may even cause the food itself to turn bad.

- Store oils, fats and oily foods like cheeses and shelled nuts in the refrigerator. This will help to slow down the process of oxidation which turns them rancid.

- Vitamin C, thiamin, riboflavin and folic acid all decay quickly in air. Once vegetables are harvested, the damaged tissues release an enzyme which starts to destroy the vitamin C. Blanching inhibits the enzyme, which is why freezing fresh vegetables is much better than keeping them unfrozen and eating them many days later.

- Vegetables lose around 70 per cent of their folic acid content within three days if they are stored in daylight. Store vegetables in the refrigerator until you are ready to use them, or freeze them straightaway.

- Store grains and cereals whole and in a dry, cool place.

- Cooking is generally harmful to the nutrients in food.

However it also changes starches, proteins and some vitamins into accessible forms for us, as well as releasing nutrients in some foods which are otherwise bound in, like the amino acid tryptophan in cornmeal. Cooking is necessary for other foods to destroy toxic substances, such as those found in soya beans and kidney beans. Cooking also makes some foods, like meat, palatable to eat. However, there are ways in which you can reduce the nutrient loss in foods during the cooking process.

- Pressure cooking is perhaps the best way to reduce nutrient loss. Invest in a non-aluminium pressure cooker which, because of the reduced cooking times, will also reduce energy consumption and therefore the size of your fuel bills.

- After pressure cooking, steaming and microwave cooking are the next healthiest options. Buying a steamer is obviously a lot cheaper than a microwave oven! Further down the list are:

  Boiling

  Grilling

  Stir-frying (at high temperature where the fat seals in the nutrients)

  Sautéing

  Deep frying

- If you cook with fat don't let it become so hot that it starts to smoke. At this temperature the essential fatty acid, linoleic acid is destroyed immediately.

- Fats which have been used for cooking once must be discarded since the linoleic acid and vitamins A and C will have been lost.

- If you boil food, do so for the minimum amount of time and then use the water for stock afterwards. The fragile water-soluble vitamins, as well as some minerals, leach into cooking water, which is why soups are so nutritious.

- Don't add bicarbonate of soda to cooking water, even if you see it recommended for cooking pulses. It destroys valuable B vitamins.

- Prepare food immediately before cooking. Remember that vitamin C is destroyed once cells are damaged in vegetables – and for the same reason try not to chop them too finely. Scrubbing vegetables is better than peeling them.

- Once prepared, immerse the vegetables in ready boiling water straightaway.

- Use pans with close-fitting lids and avoid copper pans which encourage oxidation and vitamin C loss.
- Once food is cooked, eat it straightaway. Keeping it warm will only result in further nutrient loss, which is why eating out too frequently may be less than healthy for you.

If you lead a hectic lifestyle, and consider that you don't have time for some of the advice given above, think again. The life you lead is totally dependent on a good nutritional support system – without which you're just running on empty. And you can only do that for so long. Shopping regularly for fresh foods can appear to present a problem – if you don't attach a very high priority to it. But just think: no sensible person buys a Rolls-Royce then tries to run it on two star petrol! It's the same with your body – the better the fuel, the better the performance you'll receive.

I've heard that plants contain natural chemicals which cause cancer, so nothing's really safe to eat, is it?

Yes, some plants certainly do produce chemicals to defend themselves against fungi, insects and animal predators. Consider the cabbage. It contains 49 natural pesticides and metabolites, many of which may be cancer-causing or cancer-promoting! Actually, it's been estimated that there are between 5000 and 10,000 natural pesticides and associated breakdown products in our diets. And we eat about 1.5 grams of them every day. But wait! Before you decide to give up eating for good, consider this. Even though people who eat cabbages are certainly taking in all the natural pesticides the cabbage uses to defend itself, those same people actually have a *greatly reduced* risk of getting cancer. Further, research shows that cabbage may actually retard existing cancers from spreading (metastasis). So what's going on? Simply this. *Nothing works in isolation.* A naturally healthy diet contains more than enough life-protecting nutrients – and other factors – to block the effect of minor plant toxins. So don't give up on the cabbage!

Do I have to follow the measurements given?

The more accurate you can be with your measurements, the better the system will work for you. To make things as easy as possible, most of the foods are listed in common measurements (a cup, a slice, and so on). Remember, we want you to eat as widely as possible. Do you know what the prime cause of malnutrition is? Most people in the West often erroneously believe that it's lack of food, but that's not true. The principal cause of malnutrition is lack of *variety*. A monotonous diet is a dangerous diet. So choose your food as widely as possible!

How accurate are the numbers?

As accurate as we can make them – of course. In practice, this means that we've used food values collected from the world's leading authorities for our calculations. The major variable is, inevitably, the quality and freshness of the food concerned (see above). However, let's also realize that men and women don't 'live by numbers alone'. At the end of the day, the most important function the LifePoints and RiskPoints figures serve is to awaken in you your own instinctive sense for a healthy diet. And that's the best possible use for the LifePoints Diet. We don't want you to be a slave to the numbers, we want you to use them to educate and liberate!

Can't I just subtract the RiskPoints from the LifePoints to produce one simple number?

In a word, no. When we were first developing the system, we tried to achieve this. But because they are essentially two completely different measures of a food's worth, it is not possible to combine them meaningfully. However, we think having two numbers is actually superior to one. This is why: one number tells you very little about the good and bad ingredients in a foodstuff. It doesn't allow you to make a mental picture of that food, nor does it allow you to see how and where that food might fit into your diet. Having two index numbers allows you to get more of a *feel* for the food concerned – which is what we want. When you've used the system for a day or two, you'll see what we mean.

What happens if I exceed my daily RiskPoints?

You'll get an official warning – do it again and we'll come round and wire your jaws shut! (That's a joke, by the way.) Look, we don't want you to feel that the LifePoints Diet depends on guilt in order to work, because it doesn't. Remember that your first priority is to choose *good* food to eat. And that's *fun!* Don't feel dejected if you exceed your RiskPoints limit from time to time, that's life. And in all probability, you won't drop dead! However, it's a strong indication that you're not eating the healthiest diet you could. Just try to get those RiskPoints down gradually . . . It may take some time to reeducate your tastebuds, particularly if you're used to a high-fat diet. The LifePoints system is a tool, use it as you would any other to achieve your success over a period of time. And remember: 'Success by the inch is a cinch – by the yard, it's hard!'

If I hit 100 daily LifePoints, does it guarantee that I've got all my recommended daily allowances?

No, we don't want you to hit 100 LifePoints and then sit back. As explained above, people vary widely, and recommended daily allowances (RDAs) are only generalizations. One of the most dangerous aspects of RDAs is to give people a false sense of security that they're 'well nourished'. RDAs are, in reality, 'best guesses' by a panel of government officials. When the US Department of Agriculture released its 'dietary pyramid', this is what the eminent nutritional authority Walter C. Willett, of the Harvard School of Public Health, had to say about it in *Science* magazine: 'Inevitably, such a document represents a mix of well-supported findings, educated guesses, and political compromises with powerful economic interests such as the dairy and meat industries.'[58]

Another hopeless problem with RDAs is that they're entirely impossible for ordinary people to use. Just adding up your daily food intake for *one* nutrient is difficult enough . . . but when you have to cope with a dozen or more, and watch your fat, and calories, and endlessly juggle your daily menu to make sure you hit all your RDAs – forget it! Ultimately, trying to follow any RDA system leads to one thing only (apart, that is, from madness!): pills. That's the only way you can *guarantee* that you're getting 100 per cent of the recommended daily intake for specific vitamins and minerals. And as we've already seen (under beta-carotene on page 53), pills are not a substitute for a healthy diet. The RDA approach implies that a certain (guestimated) level of nutrition is all you need to bother with. Increasingly, this assumption is being challenged. The LifePoints system goes way beyond RDAs. By showing you the good, high-nutrient foods, and steering you away from the empty or hazardous foods, you're getting the big picture. Eating a high-quality diet is far more important than worrying whether your vitamin C consumption is 55 grams or 60 grams. And that's what LifePoints can do for you.

How can I put together meals and recipes using LifePoints?

Easily! Remember, go for variety. Choose from all of the first four groups. When you've chosen a food from one group, go to another for your next food choice. As far as recipes are concerned, we'd like you to try *The Lifepoints Cookbook*, which shows you just how easy it is to produce delicious food and meals using the system. And it gives you over 150 quick, easy and economical recipes, too!

I really go to pieces at Christmas and other special occasions.

We know – these occasions are full of family and social pressures and the appeal of traditional foods. That's why we wrote *The Lifepoints Cookbook*, which has plenty of ideas for you to consider for celebrations and entertaining.

What should I do when I feel weak-willed and want to eat something with a no-no RiskPoint number?

Choose something else! There are plenty of foods with respectable LifePoints numbers and zero or little RiskPoints. Remember – you're in control! You eat what *you* want to eat. The LifePoints system is all about taking charge of your own diet. If you want to choose bad food, then that's your decision – we're not going to nag you. But here's a tip: immediately you sense that feeling, take out a notepad and write down exactly what you want to do, and put its RiskPoints number beside it in BIG FIGURES. Now look at what you have written. Your inclination to eat that food is guaranteed to diminish.

I always start diets but then get fed up cooking two meals – one for myself and another for my family.

This is a really common problem, and a difficult one too. Since preparing two sets of meals is almost impossible to do for any length of time, you must sit down with your family and explain to them the LifePoints system. Then tell them that it is difficult to make two meals and that this has, in the past, caused you many problems with diets. If they're worth their salt, they will come up with a number of ideas that may help share and solve this problem. They may decide that they want to eat healthily, too – or someone might even volunteer to help you with the food!

I'm a fast eater. When I finish my first serving, my family isn't even halfway through theirs, so I usually take another serving just to keep them company. I know this has caused a lot of my weight problems, but how can I slow down?

There are a number of simple, unobtrusive little techniques you can use to help you eat more slowly.

- Don't cut your food into pieces all at once (if it needs cutting). Instead, cut one bite-sized piece at a time, eat it then cut the next piece.
- Take a fork full of food, then put your fork down on the side of your plate while you chew that mouthful. Don't pick up the next forkful until you have swallowed the first.
- Buy a set of cloth napkins and use one at each meal. Wipe your mouth frequently during the meal to help slow you down.
- Take a slow, deep breath in and out between each mouthful of food. This will take the hurry out of eating as well as keep you relaxed.
- With all of this slow eating, you might think your food will go cold. Warm your plate before serving to prevent this. Also, take small portions of food so that the rest remains in the hot serving dish.

I use a lot of oil and fat in cooking and I've got used to the flavour. What is a good substitute for all this fat?

Cut the fat in cooking to an absolute minimum. Ignore the fat included in the recipes you use and, when it seems essential, try cutting the amount listed in half.

- Blend a little tomato, yeast extract or tandoori paste with 2 fl oz (60 ml) water and pour into your pan. Place over a high flame and, when the liquid bubbles, add your vegetables and stir frequently. This is what we call the 'New Sauté' method (see page 150), the liquid replaces the fat normally used in a sauté. You will be surprised at how tasty this is.

- Try the *LifePoints Cookbook*!

I have a really sweet tooth that always gets the better of me. What can I do to stop myself eating sweet things?

There's nothing at all wrong with eating sweet foods such as fresh fruit. Use LifePoints to find the best! But as far as puddings and desserts are concerned, then a sweet tooth is really a bully that always wants to have its own way. You will have to turn it gradually into a more respectable creature. Start by depriving your sweet tooth, a little at a time, of what it wants. Instead of a chocolate bar, eat some dried figs or raisins. Instead of sugary tea or coffee, drink it unsugared with a piece of sugarless oat cake to give you slow-release energy. Next, try re-training your sweet tooth to become a sour tooth. The flavours are equally strong, but the effects are wonderfully different. Every time you want a sweet 'injection', chew on a wedge of lemon, take a sip of cider vinegar in water, or eat a gherkin. Finally, give yourself time to break the sweet habit. If you have one or two bad days, don't give up. Keep going and you will succeed.

ON YOUR MARKS FOR THE LIFEPOINTS KICK-START!

Now we'd like to get your engine revved up for the Kick-Start – a seven-day action plan which will show you how simple, effective and enjoyable it can be to eat a diet high in LifePoints, low in RiskPoints and bursting with flavour and appeal! Read the plan, then browse through the menus, exercises and recipes. You can begin today or you can plan to start within the next few days. And later on, we'll give you more guidance on how to progress from the Kick-Start to the longer-term LifeStyle plan.

Each day of the Kick-Start provides you with over 200 LifePoints and approximately 75 RiskPoints – a very healthy profile indeed. This lets you experience the immediate impact of a reduction in high-RiskPoints foods. For some people, such as those with high cholesterol, this diet will have a significant effect on their cholesterol levels. However, should you perceive that a RiskPoints rating of 100 per day is more suitable to you, then use the listings to alter the menus described and be assured that you will still benefit greatly from the Kick-Start, as a 100 RiskPoints rating is still well below that of a 'normal' menu!

We don't think you will go hungry on the LifePoints Diet. There are three hefty meals each day and two snacks. In addition, as you can see from the listings in Part Five, there are dozens of foods you can add which will boost your LifePoints without adding RiskPoints. In fact, we think you are rather more likely to want *less* food! This is fine, just reduce the servings by one half or quarter and adjust the ratings accordingly. As you can see, even halved, you will still achieve the ideal of 100 or more LifePoints.

Like everything about LifePoints, the Kick-Start is simple and effective. So open your pantry and start!

THE FIRST WEEK
DAY ONE

Here's What to Eat!

- Choose one Breakfast from the seven breakfast menus listed.
- Choose one Morning Snack from the seven morning snacks listed.
- Choose one Lunch from the seven lunch menus listed.
- Choose one Afternoon Snack from the seven afternoon snacks listed.
- Choose one Dinner from the seven dinner menus listed.

Here's How To Exercise!

- Perform any six of the Kick-Start Stretches
- Walk One Mile.

You may be one of those people who have never exercised in your life, but you can start now, no matter what your age. Exercise begins to benefit you *immediately*, with the benefits mounting the longer you stick with it. We have provided 18 Kick-Start Stretches which help to mobilize and invigorate your body. Read through the descriptions of them (page 100) and then choose any six and perform them. You may stick with these same six throughout the week or do all of them in any combination during the course of the week. Try to enjoy these movements and make note of the effect they have on your mobility and sense of well-being throughout the day. You may notice fewer headaches, for instance, or an improvement in posture, skin tone or sleeping patterns. Perform your six movements any time of day that is convenient to you, although morning is usually considered the best time as the movements then offer greatest benefit.

Walking is an excellent form of exercise for all ages and most levels of fitness and physical condition. Because it uses the large muscles in your legs, it has maximum benefit for least cardio-respiratory effort. Your whole body benefits, not just your legs, especially if you walk briskly and with a slight swing to your arms. The benefits will be undercut if you have to pound along hard city streets, so try to find a park or unpaved lane to enjoy and become acquainted with. As with the Stretches, choose a time of day for your walk that is convenient and most enjoyable to you.

Today, Day One of the Kick-Start, pick a turning-point destination that is one-half mile from your home, or trace a route that will bring you round in a circle. You could also walk the full mile to a specific destination and then catch a bus home. Use a local map to determine the distance or guestimate a mile as being 10–12 city 'blocks'. Now put on your most comfortable shoes and go! Here are the only guidelines you need remember as you walk:

- Walk as briskly as you can without losing your breath. You should be able to talk or sing as you walk without feeling breathless or in any way uncomfortable. You may puff a tiny bit, but if you can't talk then slow down.
- Walk with an even gait and a slight swing to your arms. Humans are *meant* to walk so try to look like one of the athletic, agile creatures we once were. Visualize how you look to others at this moment and try to stand a bit taller and straighter, lift your chin and stop frowning.
- Walking needs air: breathe deeply in and out to exercise fully while you move. As you breathe in, imagine all the health and fitness rushing into your body. As you breathe out, imagine all the flab, the excess, the ill-health being pushed out of your body for ever.

That's all on walking for today, more tomorrow!

Here's What You Should Think About!

Today, write in your diet diary:

- Everything that you eat
- How much you weigh

We ask you to weigh yourself today, again at the end of the week and then once each week during the first three months of the diet, just to keep track of your success. Scales are not a critical part of the LifePoints Diet, in fact, you don't need to have any in the house. Many places, such as health clinics or chemist shops, have high-quality scales which you can use when you need to.

- What exercise do you take each week and for how long do you exercise?

Describing the exercise you do and the length of time you spend doing it is important because we want you to be able to set targets and goals for fitness a little later on. Right now, just be straightforward and give a clear answer.

DAY TWO

Here's What To Eat!
- Choose one Breakfast from the seven breakfast menus listed.
- Choose one Morning Snack from the seven morning snacks listed.
- Choose one Lunch from the seven lunch menus listed.
- Choose one Afternoon Snack from the seven afternoon snacks listed.
- Choose one Dinner from the seven dinner menus listed.

Here's How To Exercise!
- Perform any six of the Kick-Start Stretches
- Walk One Mile.

Today, Day Two of the Kick-Start, make any amendments you wish to your practice, your route or the time of day you take your walk. Certainly, do take your spouse, a friend or the dog but only if they will accompany you in the same spirit so that you do not feel held back, dragged down or disinclined. Just one thing more to do today: note in your diary how long it takes you to Walk One Mile.

Here's What You Should Think About!
Record everything you eat today. Also, we would like you to look through the listing of foods in this book, which give a representative selection of foodstuffs. A very comprehensive listing of

well over a thousand foods is available in our book *LifePoints*. Remember we said that LifePoints helps you rediscover your instincts about food? This will be accomplished most quickly by studying the lists at the same time as you alter your diet. If you have time today, have a look through your pantry and put aside or discard those things you obviously will not be needing. But more important than that, look ahead through this week's menus and make a shopping list for what is needed. Now is your chance to try a new greengrocer or explore new shops for quality ingredients. Treat this as the first week of an adventure which will enable you to indulge in excellent food for just the cost of that surplus round your middle.

DAY THREE

Here's What To Eat!
- Choose one Breakfast from the seven breakfast menus listed.
- Choose one Morning Snack from the seven morning snacks listed.
- Choose one Lunch from the seven lunch menus listed.
- Choose one Afternoon Snack from the seven afternoon snacks listed.
- Choose one Dinner from the seven dinner menus listed.

Here's How To Exercise!
- Perform any six of the Kick-Start Stretches
- Walk One Mile.

Remember, you may use this week to try all 18 of the Kick-Start Stretches and to adjust the time of day at which you perform them. Make any relevant notes or comments in your diary. Yesterday, you noted how long it took you to Walk One Mile; today try to Walk One Mile within the same period of time.

Here's What You Should Think About!
Record everything you eat today. Also, perform a few simple tests to determine your level of fitness and jot down the results in your diary. Fitness consists of these elements:

• Endurance
Also called stamina, endurance indicates a cardio-respiratory

(heart/lung) system which allows you to use the large muscles with efficiency over a sustained period of time. It also indicates an ability to recover quickly from exertion without suffering fatigue.

To test for endurance: Run on the spot, lifting your knees high, breathing regularly.

- 1 minute or less = poor endurance
- 1–1.5 minutes = average endurance
- 2 minutes or longer = good endurance

STOP if you start to feel dizzy, sick, winded or experience any discomfort in the chest.

• Strength

Strength is the force which a muscle can produce when it contracts. Strength can be acquired either by contracting the muscles in a static position with little or no movement of the joint (isometric), or by contracting them in resistance to a weight or force while moving the joint (isotonic).

To test for strength: First test your abdominal muscles. Lie on the floor with your arms folded behind your head and *roll* up into a sitting position. Abdominal strength is:

- Poor – if you can't do it
- Average – if you can get halfway up
- Good – if you can sit up easily and do so repeatedly

Now test your arm, shoulder and chest muscles. Find a sturdy table or wall unit and stand approximately 3 feet from it. Hold onto the table edge and do press-ups against it by bringing your chest down to the table edge and lifting it away again. Keep your legs straight all the while.

- 1–3 press-ups are poor
- 4–6 press-ups are average
- 7–10 are good

• Flexibility

Flexibility is indicated by the range of movement available in the joints. Flexibility involves connective tissues, such as ligaments and tendons, and the joints themselves. Flexibility determines posture and ease of movement as well as suppleness. It is, of course, closely allied to muscle tone and the amount of elasticity your muscles display.

To test for flexibility: Sit on the floor, legs together and stretched straight in front of you. Reach for your toes without straining. Reaching:

- between the ankle and knee is poor
- just the ankle is average
- over the toes is good.

Now stretch your arms up over your head and move first one then the other in a circular swimming movement. Making:

- less than half a circle is poor
- nearly a full circle or a full circle with some discomfort is average
- a full circle with no discomfort is good.

In addition, your resting pulse is a good general indicator of how fit you are, although it obviously cannot measure strength or flexibility. Find your pulse in the side of your neck using your index and middle finger, not your thumb. Men should have a resting pulse rate of between 70–85 beats a minute and women between 75–90 beats a minute. If your resting pulse rate is past the hundred mark then you definitely need to improve your fitness, but you must avoid vigorous exercise to begin with. When you are very unfit your pulse rate increases quickly as you exert yourself, and takes longer to return to normal after exercise than that of a fit person. A fit person not only has a low pulse rate to start off with, it also stays lower for longer and quickly returns to normal after activity.

Self-awareness is perhaps the most vital element in deciding how fit you are. Most people know where their shortcomings lie. If your lack of fitness is stopping you from engaging in your favourite sport or activity, then you will know it before anyone, or any test.

DAY FOUR

Here's What To Eat!
- Choose one Breakfast from the seven breakfast menus listed.
- Choose one Morning Snack from the seven morning snacks listed.
- Choose one Lunch from the seven lunch menus listed.
- Choose one Afternoon Snack from the seven afternoon snacks listed.
- Choose one Dinner from the seven dinner menus listed.

Here's How To Exercise!
- Perform any six of the Kick-Start Stretches
- Walk One Mile.

Don't let yourself get bored: change the stretches you are doing or put on your favourite music while you do them; alter the route of your walk or take someone with you. Keep in mind that this is the start of a new way of life and stay motivated.

When walking today, keep to the same time as you did Days Two and Three. Always adhere to the safety guidelines given on Day One.

Here's What You Should Think About!
Record everything you eat today. Also, make a list in your diary of:

- any serious or chronic ailments you suffer from
- any minor or recurring ailments you suffer from
- any patterns of depression, fatigue or moodiness you endure.

DAY FIVE

Here's What To Eat!
- Choose one Breakfast from the seven breakfast menus listed.
- Choose one Morning Snack from the seven morning snacks listed.
- Choose one Lunch from the seven lunch menus listed.
- Choose one Afternoon Snack from the seven afternoon snacks listed.
- Choose one Dinner from the seven dinner menus listed.

Here's How To Exercise!

- Perform any six of the Kick-Start Stretches
- Walk One Mile.

Today, try to reduce the length of time it takes you to Walk One Mile by one minute.

Here's What You Should Think About!

Record everything you eat today. Also, begin to plan your menu for next week – it is useful to start with breakfast and the morning snack. First, decide which of the breakfasts you have tried most suits you and amend it if you wish *to make it suit you more precisely*: make it more or less filling, replace one sort of fruit with another or alter the portion sizes, for example. Decide what you really enjoy, then use the food listings to work out the LifePoints and RiskPoints for the foods you have chosen. (For a listing of over a thousand foods, see our book *LifePoints*) Then it is simply a process of 'tweaking': amending until the menu is the meal you want to eat with low RiskPoints and high LifePoints to keep you well nourished. We have found that most people enjoy more or less the same breakfast every morning and so one good menu is enough for this meal. If this is not the case for you, then go ahead and devise two or three more. Actually write them out on index cards, show their LifePoints and RiskPoints totals and store them away until you need them. Now move on to the morning snack.

Again, it is a case of reworking a snack idea until it suits you and your situation precisely but healthily. Some people have a very definite preference for a sweet snack, others for a liquid snack and still others could go ahead and have their lunch at eleven o'clock in the morning! It really is up to you. But let us remind you here of some basic guidelines:

- Try not to exceed 100 RiskPoints per day and aim to acquire at least 100 LifePoints each day.
- Try to avoid double-zero foods such as sugar, jams, tea and coffee, and alcohol. They may not add to your RiskPoints but neither do they add to your LifePoints or your health.
- It doesn't matter which meal you eat at what time of day; it does matter that you *do not go hungry* and that you aim to *eat a great variety* of foods every day.

Write down several morning snack menus on index cards, with their LifePoints and RiskPoints ratings, and put them with the other cards.

DAY SIX

Here's What To Eat!
- Choose one Breakfast from the seven breakfast menus listed.
- Choose one Morning Snack from the seven morning snacks listed.
- Choose one Lunch from the seven lunch menus listed.
- Choose one Afternoon Snack from the seven afternoon snacks listed.
- Choose one Dinner from the seven dinner menus listed.

Here's How to Exercise!
- Perform any six of the Kick-Start Stretches
- Walk One Mile.

Change your selection of stretches if it suits you. Walk One Mile in the same time you walked it yesterday.

Here's What You Should Think About!
Record everything you eat today. Then, tackle Lunch and the Afternoon Snack: decide which of those you have eaten this week most suit you, amend them and record them in detail on index cards along with their ratings. Lunch, especially, can be a challenging meal to create menus for. So often it is a business or canteen lunch on offer and it can, at first, seem difficult to avoid the fat traps these types of meals present. Let us reassure you: even the most dire canteen or café offers a salad these days. Have that and a baked potato without butter and you won't go hungry or clock up huge numbers of RiskPoints. Also, you will get familiar with high-LifePoints foods within the next week or so – if you haven't already. We have said that LifePoints helps you rediscover your instinct for good food and this becomes apparent very early on when you find yourself in a situation with few food choices. If you make your own lunches, planning menus is much easier and more certain; if you rely on restaurants and canteens then use this time, today, to read through the food listings once again to familiarize yourself with high-LifePoints foods.

DAY SEVEN

Here's What To Eat!
- Choose one Breakfast from the seven breakfast menus listed.
- Choose one Morning Snack from the seven morning snacks listed.
- Choose one Lunch from the seven lunch menus listed.
- Choose one Afternoon Snack from the seven afternoon snacks listed.
- Choose one Dinner from the seven dinner menus listed.

Here's How To Exercise!
- Perform any six of the Kick-Start Stretches
- Walk One Mile.

Try to secure the time of day you perform your stretches and take your walk. Schedule it in if necessary. For the next month, it is important that you do not forego this exercise programme. One month is long enough for most people to feel that exercise has become a part of their life. You may go through further stages of amending your route and your practice, but hopefully you will put time aside each day for exercise of some sort. We will talk more about exercise later (see page 155), but we trust that you have noted some benefit or difference to yourself from the exercises you have performed this week. Please record these perceptions in your diary.

Here's What You Should Think About!
Record everything you eat today. Also, weigh yourself and make a note of it. Then, plan the menus for next week and compile a shopping list. You have done most of the work for breakfast, lunch and snacks; it remains for you to work out your menus for next week's dinners. Some guidelines:

- Use the recipes included in this book, or in *The Lifepoints Cookbook* to make meals that are already assessed for Life-Points and RiskPoints.
- Don't make hard work out of this! Just like everyone else, use your leftovers for lunch the next day or prepare meals in advance and freeze them. We have compiled a list of tips to help you keep it all very easy, see page 150.

- Start simple, then, when you feel at ease with choosing and preparing your foods for maximum LifePoints, begin to experiment with meals that you find more adventurous. Then again, you might not like adventure in your meals! Remember, LifePoints is a tool for you to use to make the diet that suits you.

THE KICK-START MENUS

Breakfasts

Breakfast One
1 serving 40% Bran Flakes or Raisin Bran with skimmed milk
1 banana or 1 cup fresh blackberries or raspberries
1 glass fresh orange juice
1 cup tea or coffee with milk
✗ RiskPoints 16
✔ LifePoints 59

Breakfast Two
porridge made with skimmed milk
1 toasted crumpet spread with yeast extract
half a cantaloupe melon
1 glass pineapple juice
1 cup tea or coffee with milk
✗ RiskPoints 20
✔ LifePoints 50

Breakfast Three
1 slice toast spread with yeast extract
half tin of baked beans served over it
1 small bowl stewed prunes
1 banana
1 glass fresh orange juice
1 cup tea or coffee with milk
✗ RiskPoints 18
✔ LifePoints 50

Breakfast Four
homemade fruit salad made from fresh or dried dates, 1 banana, dried apricots and currants

topped with skimmed milk yogurt
and ½oz toasted wheat germ
1 glass pineapple juice
1 cup tea or coffee with milk
✘ RiskPoints 17
✔ LifePoints 53

Breakfast Five
Grape Nuts cereal with skimmed milk
half a cantaloupe melon
1 glass fresh orange juice
1 cup tea or coffee with milk
✘ RiskPoints 15
✔ LifePoints 54

Breakfast Six
1 bowl Rice Krispies or Corn Flakes with skimmed milk
1 plain bagel spread with yeast extract
1 banana
1 glass fresh orange juice
1 cup tea or coffee with milk
✘ RiskPoints 17
✔ LifePoints 64

Breakfast Seven
1 bowl fortified oatflakes cereal (i.e. Common Sense) with
skimmed milk
1 plain, toasted crumpet spread with yeast extract
1 apple
1 glass apple juice
1 cup tea or coffee with milk
✘ RiskPoints 17
✔ LifePoints 58

Morning Snacks
AM Snack One
toasted crumpet spread with yeast extract
1 glass vegetable juice cocktail
✘ RiskPoints 2
✔ LifePoints 24

AM Snack Two
1 pitta bread filled with Bean Pâté (page 120) and alfalfa sprouts
1 glass vegetable juice cocktail
✘ RiskPoints 1
✔ LifePoints 28

AM Snack Three
3–4 spears steamed asparagus with low-fat French dressing
1 breadstick
1 glass carrot juice
✘ RiskPoints 4
✔ LifePoints 24

AM Snack Four
1 bagel (plain, poppy seed, sesame seed or onion) spread with
boiled, mashed sweet chestnuts garnished with salt, pepper and
cress
1 glass vegetable juice cocktail
✘ RiskPoints 2
✔ LifePoints 22

AM Snack Five
1 handful each soft-dried apricots, figs and gingko nuts
1 glass vegetable juice cocktail
✘ RiskPoints 3
✔ LifePoints 28

AM Snack Six
1 carrot, cut into sticks
1 stalk celery, cut into sticks
approximately 3oz Bean Pâté (page 120)
1 glass tomato juice
✘ RiskPoints 0
✔ LifePoints 27

AM Snack Seven
1 bagel (plain, poppy seed, sesame seed or onion)
1 cup sauerkraut
1 glass vegetable juice cocktail
✘ RiskPoints 2
✔ LifePoints 26

Lunches
Lunch One
baked potato filled with baked beans (no butter)
mixed vegetable salad with low-fat French dressing
1 apple
1 glass pineapple juice
1 slice banana bread (made with margarine)
✘ RiskPoints 19
✔ LifePoints 40

Lunch Two
1 slice olive pizza (no cheese)
mixed vegetable salad with low-fat Thousand Island dressing
half a cantaloupe melon
1 glass fresh orange juice
1 slice raisin bread
✘ RiskPoints 16
✔ LifePoints 41

Lunch Three
1 vegetable burger in a bun with condiments
mixed vegetable salad with low-fat French dressing
1 glass pineapple juice
1 bowl fresh raspberries or blackberries with crispbread or ricecakes (these may be crumbled over the fruit)
✘ RiskPoints 20
✔ LifePoints 41

Lunch Four
1 whole pitta bread stuffed with mixed vegetable salad with low-fat French dressing and 1 falafel
half a cantaloupe melon
1 glass fresh orange juice
1 cinnamon raisin bagel
✘ RiskPoints 15
✔ LifePoints 46

Lunch Five
1 slice toast spread with yeast extract served with half tin baked beans

1 medium potato, steamed grilled or steamed mushrooms (½ cup)
1 apple
1 glass apple juice
1 slice banana bread (made with margarine)
✘ RiskPoints 20
✔ LifePoints 45

Lunch Six
vegetable cutlet (no nuts)
mixed vegetable salad with low-fat French dressing
1 banana
1 glass fresh orange juice
1 cinnamon-raisin bagel
✘ RiskPoints 18
✔ LifePoints 41

Lunch Seven
spaghetti with tomato and mushroom sauce
mixed vegetable salad with low-fat Italian dressing
1 orange
1 glass pineapple juice
1 scone
✘ RiskPoints 19
✔ LifePoints 44

Afternoon Snacks
PM Snack One
1 bagel (plain, poppy seed, sesame seed or onion)
1 sliced tomato
sliced cucumber or dill pickle
1 glass vegetable juice cocktail
✘ RiskPoints 3
✔ LifePoints 21

PM Snack Two
1 handful dried figs
1 glass carrot juice
✘ RiskPoints 2
✔ LifePoints 20

PM Snack Three
1 slice wholewheat toast spread with yeast extract
1 glass tomato juice
✘ RiskPoints 2
✔ LifePoints 20

PM Snack Four
1 handful soft dried apricots
1 handful soft dried pears
1 glass orange juice
✘ RiskPoints 2
✔ LifePoints 21

PM Snack Five
1 slice granary bread (or 3 ricecakes)
spread with Bean Pâté (page 120)
1 glass tomato juice
✘ RiskPoints 2
✔ LifePoints 20

PM Snack Six
1 pitta bread filled with
sliced artichoke hearts with low-fat French dressing
1 glass vegetable juice cocktail
✘ RiskPoints 3
✔ LifePoints 20

PM Snack Seven
1 large spear steamed broccoli
covered with sprouted mung beans
dressed with low-fat French dressing
1 glass tomato juice
✘ RiskPoints 3
✔ LifePoints 21

Dinners
Dinner One
start with half a cantaloupe melon
spaghetti with Sun-Dried Tomato Bolognaise Sauce (page 145)
mixed vegetable salad with low-fat French dressing
1 slice Italian, pumpernickel or rye bread

after which 1 piece Fruit and Cereal Snack Bar (page 127)
✘ RiskPoints 25
✔ LifePoints 100

Dinner Two
start with Cream of Mushroom Soup (page 125)
Marinated Steak and Mushrooms with Roast Potatoes (page 132)
steamed chicory greens
steamed carrots
after which fresh raspberries or blackberries
✘ RiskPoints 19
✔ LifePoints 111

Dinner Three
start with Creamed Vegetable Soup (page 126)
Bean and Mushroom Cannelloni (page 119)
All-Colour Salad (page 115) with low-fat Italian dressing
after which a plate of fresh grapes
✘ RiskPoints 11
✔ LifePoints 112

Dinner Four
start with Asparagus in Garlic Orange Sauce (page 117)
Wild Rice Risotto (page 146) with
Spiced Garden Beans (page 142)
steamed broccoli
after which Bean Pâté (page 120) on matzos, ricecakes or
crispbreads
✘ *RiskPoints* 7
✔ *LifePoints* 112

Dinner Five
start with Melon and Apricot Smoothie (page 134)
Red Hot Vegetable Curry (page 139)
Spiced Kidney Bean Ragout (page 142)
over steamed rice
after which fresh lychees
✘ *RiskPoints* 7
✔ *LifePoints* 105

Dinner Six
start with Garlic Bread (page 128)
Lasagne Bolognaise (page 131)
Beans and Greens Salad (page 120) with low-fat Thousand Island dressing
after which a plate of fresh or dried dates
✘ RiskPoints 20
✔ LifePoints 111

Dinner Seven
start with a glass of pineapple juice
Beefless Stroganoff (page 121)
over steamed rice
with steamed spinach and
Heart of Gold Roasted Pumpkin (page 130)
after which Apple and Raspberry Pie (page 116)
✘ RiskPoints 10
✔ LifePoints 123

THE KICK-START STRETCHES
The exercises that follow are all easy to learn, easy to perform and gradually, but definitely, effective in improving your suppleness, strength and mobility. But more than this, they all chip away at the collection of poor movement, posture and breathing habits you may have been nursing along for years. Like any habit which stops you from getting the most out of your life, these habits can be replaced.

By gently introducing a few of these movements into your daily life, you will begin to sit taller, walk more sprightly, sleep more soundly, digest more easily, move with less pain, work with more energy. After a few weeks, you won't quite believe that you used to tell the time by your mid-morning twinges or your five o'clock tension headache. Pick six of these exercises and perform them daily during this Kick-Start week.

Ringing the Bell
Stand or sit tall and raise both arms over your head. Look either straight in front of you or up at your hands. Now stretch one hand up and past the other as though you were grasping a rope. Stretch the second hand up past the first in the same manner.

Continue in this way and establish a very rhythmic movement – as if you were pulling a bell rope. Perform this stretch 12–20 times and breathe in as you pull with one hand, out as you pull with the other. Lower your arms and rest.

WHY? This movement stimulates circulation to your upper body and encourages large, deep breaths. It also stretches your spine and upper body so that you feel more aligned after your night's sleep. You'll feel slightly taller and very much more alert.

Shoulder Shimmy

a) Stand or sit tall and relax your arms and shoulders so that they feel heavy. Now push your shoulders back as far as you can so that your chest and the front of your shoulders feels stretched. Breathe in as you do this.

b) Next, pull your shoulders forward as far as you can so that your upper back and lower neck feels stretched. Breathe out as you do this.

Repeat these two movements three or four times then move on to the next part of the shoulder shimmy.

c) Bring either one or both shoulders up in a shrug – as close to your ears as possible. Breathe in as you do this.

d) Now drop your shoulders and stretch them down as far as they will go. Breathe out as you do this.

Repeat these two movements three or four times then move on to the next part of the shoulder shimmy.

Lift either one or both shoulders in a shrug (c) as you breathe in. From that position, roll them back into the (a) position. As you breathe out, continue to roll them down into the (d) position. Begin to breathe in again as you continue to roll your shoulder forward into the (b) position. Return to the shrug position (c) and repeat this entire movement three or four times more. Then try to reverse the direction of the shimmy.

WHY? This movement releases tension in the neck and shoulder muscles and greatly improves circulation and muscle tone in that region. Breathing is also stimulated in this movement – people who suffer respiratory problems should perform it several times daily. Upper spine alignment and mobility is improved through regular use of this shimmy.

Dry Swimming

Stand or sit tall and lift one or both arms away from your sides. You may hold your arms straight or slightly bent at the elbows, whichever is most comfortable for you. Now begin to move your arms from the shoulders so that your hands trace a circle. Imagine that you are pulling yourself through water and gradually increase the size of the movement you make. Breathe slowly and deeply, just as though you were coming up out of water for air.

Repeat this movement at your own chosen speed four to twelve times. Reverse the direction of the circle – as though swimming backwards.

WHY? This movement gently builds strength and stamina. It encourages you to hold your upper spine in proper alignment while you perform a fairly strenuous movement to build the surrounding muscles. Your attention to breathing will help to improve your stamina. The muscle tone you gain in your arms, shoulders and upper back will make some of your daily tasks (lifting and carrying) much easier and it will undermine any old posture habits (like rounding your upper back) you might have. After this movement, you will feel warm and full of energy.

Oliver Twist

Stand tall in the centre of your room and spread your feet about 12 inches apart. Let your arms hang loosely by your sides and take a breath or two in and out. Now begin, gently at first, to swing your arms around, crossing in front and behind your body – like you did as a child. You may gradually increase the speed and/or size of this movement, as you please. Perform it from side to side for one or two minutes.

WHY? This movement twists most of your spine and so helps to improve tone in those muscles that support your spine. It helps your breathing become rhythmic and deep even when you don't think about it. And, because the alignment of your spine is so important to your mood and level of vitality, this movement leaves you with a sense of elation and enthusiasm for the day ahead.

Spinal Curls

Stand tall with your feet 12 inches apart, your arms and shoulders relaxed. Now bend your knees slightly and drop your chin forward, onto your chest. Hold this briefly while you breathe in and out.

Keep your knees bent, your head resting forward and let your arms and shoulders slump forward also. You will feel a stretch somewhere in your back. Hold this position while you breathe in and out.

Next, let your arms drag you down and forward until your hands are about level with your knees. Hold this position – knees still bent, head still dropped forward – while you breathe in and out.

This part is optional – do it only if you have felt comfortable so far. Continue to curl forward until your hands nearly touch your ankles. Your knees are still bent, though probably more so than when you started, and your head must remain dropped down so that your neck muscles are relaxed. Again, hold this position while you breathe in and out.

NOTE: You may perform this curl through all four stages or just through one or two. It is your body and your choice. Do what is comfortable and you will find that, after a time, you will feel at ease progressing onto the next stage.

To come back into the upright position, simply reverse the movement. Think from the bottom of your spine and *slowly and gently* push it back into its upright position: put your waist above your pelvis, ribs above your waist, shoulders over your ribs, and finally lift your chin. Now straighten your legs and breathe slowly and deeply.

WHY? This movement stretches several groups of muscle throughout your body. Stretching is great for releasing tension, so most of the aches and pains and stiffness you woke up with will disappear after two or three of these curls. Because this movement involves almost all of your body, your overall circulation is stimulated.

Racer's Stretch

Face a wall or door and place your hands flat against it at shoulder height and about shoulder width apart. Now reach one leg straight back so that you have to bend your forward leg. Keep both sets of toes facing forward and keep both heels flat on the floor. You should feel a stretch in the calf muscle of your straight leg – the one reaching behind you.

To increase the stretch, gently pulse your body forward, towards the wall, without lifting that heel. When you are ready, repeat the movement with your legs in their opposite positions. Remember to breathe!

WHY? This stretch improves circulation to your lower legs and feet. It will help prevent problems with cold limbs and poor circulation and also adds tone to the muscles of your lower legs. Good muscle tone here supports your veins so that varicose problems are minimized. And if you spend much of the day on your feet, this stretch will be a useful antidote to fatigue – just perform it once or twice more during the day.

Persian Pelvis

Stand or sit tall and place your hands on your hips. You should literally hold onto the bony plates you can feel just below waist level. (These bones are the top of your pelvis.) Now relax your grip and tilt your pelvis so that these bones move forward and your tail-bone moves back. Now reverse the movement: the top of your pelvis moves back and your tail-bone moves forward, or under you.

If you are standing during this movement, bend your knees slightly. This will enable you to perform a larger, more definite movement.

The second part of the movement is best done in a standing position. You may lean forward slightly, or stand unsupported. In both cases, bend your knees slightly. Now think of your tail-bone and the top of your pelvis tracing a circle and move your pelvis in a round or rotating manner. This is very like a belly dance (hence the name of this exercise) and you should attempt to keep the movement relaxed and loose. Breathe regularly and keep your arms, shoulders and upper body as relaxed as possible. Circle four times in each direction and repeat this movement often during the day.

WHY? The tilting movements are excellent to relieve lower backache and may be performed in the sitting position. The rotation of the pelvis also relieves lower back pain but it has the added advantage of minimizing it in the first place – especially if you do this movement often. The rotation stimulates the functioning of your internal organs, so improving digestion, elimination and metabolism. It is good for waist and abdominal muscles and, of course, strengthens the muscles of the back. Enjoy it if you can, laugh if you like and try to perform it daily for the rest of your life.

Because the rotation also includes the lower part of your spine, this movement does create improvements in your mood and level of vitality.

Skier's Waltz

Stand facing the back of a chair and place your feet about 12 inches apart. Hold onto the back of the chair, without gripping very hard, and relax your arms and shoulders. Keep relaxed and, using the chair for balance, lift and lower your heels so that you push yourself up and down on the balls of your feet.

Repeat this movement several times. You will notice a warmth or tension creeping up the back of your legs – this is normal. When you need a break, lower your heels and bounce your knees forward, towards the chair. This part of the movement will relax the tension in your leg muscles. Repeat both parts of the movement three or four times.

WHY? The Skier's Waltz greatly improves circulation to your lower legs and feet. It is a wonderful antidote to fatigue and heaviness felt in that area and helps to prevent swelling and varicose problems. In addition, it improves muscle tone of the entire leg and into the buttocks. Good muscle tone helps to support your veins, improves mobility in your joints and improves your stamina and keeps you a nice shape. If you persevere with this movement, the tension felt as you lift and lower your heels will gradually become less significant. The movement will then begin to affect your back and you may notice that lower back discomfort is reduced.

Refreshing Footsies

This little set of movements may be done in public without getting too much of a laugh! They are best performed sitting with your body quite relaxed and comfortable. They may be done with both feet simultaneously or one foot at a time.

First, moving your foot from the ankle, stretch your heel away from you as you pull your toes and the top of your foot back towards you.

Now reverse it: stretch your toes and the top of your foot away from you as you tuck your heel back and under. Repeat these several times in a slow but definite manner – really try to increase the stretches.

Relax your foot and, still moving it from the ankle, begin to rotate it so that your toes trace a circle. Now rotate it in the opposite direction. You may notice that one foot is 'looser' than the other – this is normal, but you should try to increase the size of the circles none the less.

Repeat these movements with both feet, several times each day.

WHY? As you may have guessed, these movements also stimulate circulation to the lower legs and feet. They relieve fatigue but have the additional effect of making you feel more alert – so do them during meetings or on other soporific occasions! Varicose veins and problems with chilblains or constantly cold feet may be aided by performing these move-ments frequently on a daily basis.

Tension Zappers

Stand or sit with your spine very tall and upright. Relax your arms and shoulders and breathe deeply, in and out, three or four times. Being careful to keep your back straight, gently drop your chin forward towards your chest. You will feel a stretch in the back of your neck or at some other point in your back. Hold this position for 5–10 seconds.

Now clasp both hands behind your neck and allow your elbows to relax around your ears. Hold this position for 10–30 seconds, breathing deeply all the while. You will feel a greater sense of stretch in your neck and back due to the added weight of your arms. This may feel very strong at first and, in that case, you may wish to hold the position for a shorter period of time. As you get used to the movement, however, you will find it easier to hold the position for longer.

WHY? This movement helps to release a great deal of tension from the neck, shoulder and upper back. Often tension in these areas is chronic and causes headaches, irritability and a general preoccupation that prevents concentration. Holding the stretch while you breathe deeply releases tension, although it may at first feel slightly uncomfortable. Releasing tension will help you to avoid headaches and chronic discomfort in that area. Blood flow to your brain is improved and you may find it easier to move your head from side to side.

Armchair Twist
Sit slightly forward in a chair and straighten your back. Place both feet flat on the floor and turn your upper body to one side. Try to place one hand on the back of the chair, the other on the side or arm (if the chair has arms). Hold this twisted position for two breaths, in and out, then turn back to centre and repeat the twist in the other direction. It is important to turn your head as you twist and look as far round behind you as possible while you breathe. Repeat this two or three times each day, especially if you work in a sedentary job.

WHY? This twist helps to prevent the build up of tension in the muscles of your back, shoulders and neck. It also 'opens' your chest so that, when you get back to work, your posture is better and your breathing unimpaired. The total effect is that you become more alert and more comfortable.

'Get Off My Back' Stretch
Stand in front of a desk or cupboard and lean onto it through your hands or elbows. Step backwards so that your back is fairly straight, spread your legs about 2 feet apart and straighten your

legs also. You will be in a sort of upside-down 'L' shape and should feel that much of your body weight is being transferred through your arms and shoulders and not very much through your back and legs. Relax your neck by dropping your head down, if you like.

Now very slowly and gently bend one knee, straighten it again, bend the other knee, and straighten it also. Repeat this movement, from side to side, 4–6 times. Keep breathing deeply and slowly, and try to enjoy the feeling of movement in your pelvis and the sense of lightness in your back.

WHY? This movement helps to release tension from the lower back, hips and pelvis by literally taking the weight off those areas. In fact, the whole of your back and neck are benefited, as are the muscles in the back of your thighs. Perform this movement when you need to de-stress, catch your breath, refocus your concentration, or whenever someone or some event has been a 'pain in the back' to you!

The following movements are best performed at the end of your working day. In fact, for some people they are best done in sequence on the bed. Just push the covers aside and give yourself a total of five minutes to try them all. They conveniently finish in a reclining position, so you need only pull the covers over yourself and count to five. You'll be asleep in four!

Arm and Chest Stretch
Stand or sit tall and reach both arms up over your head. Clasp your hands together and straighten your arms as best you can. Now move both arms backwards, from your shoulders, in a gentle pulsing movement. Make sure you breathe by reciting a poem or singing along to your favourite song. Continue this pulsing movement for 30–60 seconds then lower your arms and shake them gently to relax them.

Reverse the movement by clasping your hands behind you, just over your tail-bone. Pull your shoulder blades together and gently pulse your arms up towards the ceiling for 30–60 seconds. Breathe deeply and regularly as you do so and continue to hold your back straight – do not lean forward. When you have finished, release your clasp and shake your arms once again.

WHY? This movement focuses specifically on the area around your shoulders – both front and back of your body. In the first part of the movement your upper spine is gently mobilized to rid you of stiffness, tension and poor posture. The underarm area and your pectoral (chest) muscles are also stretched, which further helps your posture and, by the way, your breathing.

The second part of the movement also frees the upper spine of tension and 'opens' the chest to improve posture and breathing. Both poor posture and shallow breathing can add to any problems you may have getting to sleep or sleeping restfully.

Diamond Hinge

Sit tall and place the soles of your feet together a comfortable distance from you so that your knees rest out to your sides. Place your hands behind you for support and lengthen your back into a straight line. Now 'hinge' your back forwards and backwards. This movement comes from your hips, not your waist, and may be quite small at first. You will feel it in your thighs and lower back. Repeat it 12–20 times, slowly and gently, and breathe evenly as you do so.

WHY? This movement relaxes the muscles of the inner thighs, buttocks and lower back. Often these muscles accumulate considerable tension during the day, which can cause backache, painful hip joints, or a general discomfort during your sleep. The hinging movement relaxes your breathing and gently stimulates the function of your abdominal organs. Indigestion, constipation and period pains are gently eased as a result. This movement is also very soothing in a mental and emotional sense as it provides you with an opportunity to 'breathe out' your worries and focus, instead, on the restful elements of your life.

Suspension Bridge

Lie on your back and slide your feet up close to your buttocks. Your feet should remain flat on the floor, about 12 inches apart, and your knees should be open to that same distance. Now relax your arms a little distance from your sides and breathe deeply three or four times. Each time you breathe out imagine all the tension rushing out of your body.

Slowly raise your tail-bone off the floor towards the ceiling. Let the rest of your spine follow, one inch at a time, until you are resting on the area of spine just between your shoulder blades. Your feet are still flat, your knees still apart. Hold this 'suspension' for one or two breaths, in and out, then slowly lower your spine onto the floor again. Start at the top of your spine and lower 1 inch at a time onto the floor until you have placed your tailbone back in its starting position. Rest here then repeat the movement two or three times more.

It is important to hold your body in a fairly straight line while you are in the lifted position. To this end, imagine that a board is supporting the back of your body. This will prevent you lowering your pelvis while you are in the suspended position – a movement that could create discomfort in your lower back.

WHY? This movement strengthens the back of your body and your thighs but, more importantly, it relieves the downward pressure of your torso into your pelvis. Spending all day in an upright position can create a feeling of compression in the lower spine. This movement turns you upside-down to a small degree and so reverses this compression. You feel 'easier' and 'freer' in the lower spine and pelvis as a result. These feelings improve your sleep and reduce mental and emotional stress.

At the same time, the front of your body, your abdomen in particular, will feel slightly stretched. This position improves the function of your abdominal organs and enhances your ability to breathe deeply and thoroughly, both of which continue the reduction of stress and tension.

Knee-to-Chest Bellows

Continue to lie flat on your back but bring both knees close to your chest and wrap your arms around them. Now hug them tightly towards you (this is the bellows position) and hold that position for two or three breaths, in and out. Keep hold of your knees but relax the hug so that you have a little more room to breathe. Rest here briefly then repeat the 'bellows' hug three more times.

If you feel like it, roll gently along your spine while you are in the bellows position – this may feel especially nice in your lower back.

WHY? The bellows movement brings a great sense of ease to the lower back and hips. So, for instance, if you suffer from a rheumatic disorder of the hips or from chronic lower backache, this movement may ease your discomfort and enable you to fall asleep more easily. In addition, holding the bellows position gives a gentle squeeze to the abdominal organs and thus encourages better function. Constipation is also minimized when this movement is performed daily.

Knee-to-Floor Twist

Lie on your back and place your feet flat on the floor quite close to your buttocks (as in the Suspension Bridge). Let your arms rest a short distance from the sides of your body and breathe deeply and easily.

On your next breath out, allow both knees to drop to one side and, at the same time, turn your face in the opposite direction. Hold this position for one or two breaths, in and out, then, on the next breath in, bring your knees and your face back to their upright, central position.

Repeat this movement to your other side.

Repeat both movements slowly, once or twice more, ensuring that you turn your face during each twist.

WHY? This movement mobilizes the whole of your spine. Your spine is crucial to your posture, nervous system and emotional state and this movement creates an overall sense of well-being. You may even find yourself sighing during this movement – a way of releasing both emotional and physical stress from your body.

The articulation of so many joints decreases tension in the muscles around the spine – from the very lower back right through to your neck. The effect is an improvement in posture, both during your sleep and in the early part of the next day. There is also a reduction in tension-related disorders such as headaches, chronic back and neck pains and chronic shoulder discomfort. This movement builds an awareness of and an improvement in your breathing patterns, which further reduces stress and increases the restfulness of your sleep.

Reclining Stretch

Lie flat on your back with your legs straight and your arms stretched over your head. Breathe deeply and evenly as you allow your feet to rest 'open', with the toes facing out to your sides. Check that your middle back is relaxing towards the floor or bed and bring your chin comfortably close to your neck.

On your next breath in, stretch while imagining one person pulling your fingers away over your head and another person pulling your toes away beyond your feet. Really exagerate this sense of stretch, hold it for 5 seconds then release the stretch as you breathe out. Breathe in and out once, then repeat the stretch as you next breathe in. During each stretch, imagine your body growing in length and pressing closely into the floor or bed. Try to enjoy this sensation before you release the stretch and relax into a heavy resting position. Repeat the stretch 4–6 times more – then pull the covers over you and allow yourself to fall asleep.

WHY? This movement is a means of getting rid of much residual tension. Because it includes all of your body, a very general, even sense of release is possible. The previous five movements have dealt with specific regions of the body but this movement allows a total body relaxation which leaves you feeling very calm, comfortable and ready to rest.

WHY WALK ONE MILE?

In addition to the Kick-Start Stretches, the LifePoints Kick-Start exercise programme is very simple: Walk One Mile.

You have seen that simple prescription repeated every day during the Kick-Start programme, and in the weeks and months ahead you will hopefully find that our challenge to Walk One Mile becomes less and less of a challenge. This is exactly as it should be and indicates that you are gaining fitness. Here are some guidelines to help you extend your walking to keep it a slight challenge and to increase your fitness through it.

- Your first goal is to Walk One Mile. You may not be able to at this stage but, provided you are medically and potentially able to achieve this goal, you can eventually with gradual and determined perseverance.
- Next try to Walk One Mile in 20 minutes. Take as long as you

need to reach this goal so that you achieve it safely and happily using the guidelines outlined on Day One.

- When you can Walk One Mile within 20 minutes then we suggest you gradually speed up your walk so that you eventually Walk One Mile within 15 minutes.

- When you can Walk One Mile in 15 minutes, then we suggest you gradually increase the length of your 'mile' until you are walking two miles in 30 minutes, approximately the same speed per mile.

- At this stage you are likely to find walking very comfortable and we advise that you use it freely, as a major mode of transport, perhaps walking up to 30 miles per week. If you wish, you may carry shopping, library books or whatever as you walk, perhaps choosing a backpack rather than a shoulder bag which would cause you to walk lopsided.

- Because walking is such a natural and usually gentle exercise it may be done daily – certainly this is ideal. However, aim for a good walk five days per week. This will allow for periods of rest and the occasional interruptions to practice which are likely.

- If and when you feel the need or inclination, extend your practice of exercise to include a sport, dance or other activity, see page 155. However, we suggest that you keep walking – every day if possible – as part of your daily routine for the rest of your life.

PART THREE: FOOD, GLORIOUS LIFEPOINTS FOOD!

We have to make an apology here. Diet food is supposed to taste incredibly boring, or to be served in incredibly small portions – and preferably both! None of these recipes are like that *at all* – so these recipes probably aren't what you were expecting!

What we *do* take delight in presenting you with is a rather wonderful collection of our own personal recipes, which we enjoy all the time. They're all new and haven't appeared anywhere else before. They're simple to make, using ingredients which you can mostly find in your local supermarkets (one or two use slightly exotic ingredients – and why not? – which you can find in your local health food store). If you like our simple but luscious taste in food, then do buy *The LifePoints Cookbook*, where you'll find a further 150 recipes to choose from. We welcome you to this collection with just one word: *Enjoy!*

All-Colour Salad

Serves 4
Preparation time: 25 minutes
✔ *LifePoints per serving: 20*
✘ *RiskPoints per serving: 5*

1 medium turnip, peeled and shredded
1 small raw beetroot, peeled and shredded
2 medium carrots, peeled and shredded
3 spring onions, finely chopped
450g (1 lb) cooked or tinned green beans
1 apple, finely chopped
1 orange, peeled, segmented and chopped, reserving juice
2 tablespoons fresh parsley, finely chopped
2 tablespoons fresh mint, finely chopped
juice and zest of 2 lemons
¼ teaspoon freshly ground black pepper
pinch of salt
1 tablespoon tahini

85g (3oz) (approximately 8 inner leaves) cos lettuce
55g (2oz) dandelion leaves

Toss all the vegetables, fruit and herbs together in a large salad bowl. Pour the juice and zest of the lemons into a jug or jam jar and add the pepper, salt and tahini. Stir or shake well. Serve the salad into brightly coloured bowls lined with the lettuce and dandelion leaves. Pour a little of the dressing over and serve.

Apple and Raspberry Pie

Serves 6
Preparation time: 55 minutes
✔ *LifePoints per serving: 33*
✘ *RiskPoints per serving: 6*

1 × recipe for New Pastry (see page 134)
3 tablespoons plain flour
1 teaspoon ground cinnamon
½ teaspoon ground cloves
¼ teaspoon ground nutmeg
450g (1lb) cooking apples, peeled, cored and sliced
450g (1lb) fresh or frozen raspberries
juice of ½ lemon

Preheat the oven to 190°C/375°F/Gas Mark 5. Prepare the pastry and reserve about one quarter of it. Press the remainder into a deep 23cm (9 inch) pie dish. Mix the flour and spices together in a small bowl and dredge the apples in this mixture. Arrange the apple slices in the pie dish and turn the raspberries and their juice over the apples. Sprinkle any remaining flour mixture over the berries; pour the lemon juice over all. Flour a board and roll the reserved pastry into a round; carefully lift this and place over the pie. Seal the edges, prick the top with a fork and bake for 35 minutes. Leave to cool on a wire rack, then slice and serve.

NOTE: You may crumble the reserved pastry over the top of the pie, instead of rolling it, if you wish. In this case, you may need to reduce the baking time by 5–10 minutes.

Asparagus in Garlic Orange Sauce

Serves 4
Preparation time: 35 minutes
✔ *LifePoints per serving: 19*
✘ *RiskPoints per serving: 0*

1 bulb garlic
180ml (6 fl oz) carrot juice
1 tablespoon arrowroot (kuzu)
juice and zest of 3 oranges
450g (1lb) asparagus, trimmed
freshly ground black pepper, to taste

Break the bulb of garlic into cloves but do not peel them yet. Drop the cloves into a small pan of boiling water and simmer until just tender – 5–7 minutes, depending on their size. Lift from the water and carefully peel the cloves, scraping the tender flesh into a small saucepan. Add the carrot juice to the garlic and whisk together over a medium heat. Measure the arrowroot into a cup and pour a little of the orange juice over it. Stir to make a cream. Add this to the hot garlic and carrot mixture and keep stirring as you add the remainder of the orange juice and the zest. The sauce should thicken nicely. Add water or more orange juice if desired.

Steam the asparagus (with the thick ends in the water if possible) until just tender. Turn onto warmed plates, pour a little of the sauce over and season to taste.

NOTE: you may substitute tomato juice for the carrot juice, in which case adjust the LifePoints to 18. RiskPoints are still 0.

Baked Lemon Tempeh

Serves 4
Preparation time: 1 hour
✔ *LifePoints per serving: 39*
✘ *RiskPoints per serving: 23*

2 × 225g (8oz) blocks tempeh, defrosted
4 teaspoons yeast extract

juice and zest of 4 lemons
100g (4oz) fresh parsley, finely chopped
3 spring onions, finely chopped
2 tablespoons fresh ginger, grated

Preheat the oven to 180°C/350°F/Gas Mark 4. Slice the tempeh blocks diagonally in half then turn each half onto its long edge and slice into three triangles. When you have sliced all the tempeh (12 triangles), spread one side of each piece with a little yeast extract. Arrange 6 triangles in a casserole, spread-side-down, onto the bottom of the dish. Mix the lemon zest, chopped parsley, onions and grated ginger together in a mixing bowl. Sprinkle this mixture over the tempeh in the casserole. Arrange the remaining tempeh triangles over the parsley mixture, placing the side spread with yeast extract uppermost. Pour the lemon juice over the tempeh, cover the casserole tightly and bake for 40 minutes. Remove the cover and bake for a final 5 minutes then serve onto warmed plates with steamed wild rice and pumpkin.

Baked Potato with Broad Bean and Broccoli Filling

Serves 4
Preparation time: 1 hour 15 minutes
✔ *LifePoints per serving: 46*
✘ *RiskPoints per serving: 3*

4 large potatoes, scrubbed
450g (1lb) broccoli, cut into florets
225g (8oz) broad beans
1 teaspoon yeast extract.
60ml (2fl oz) water
1 medium onion, thinly sliced
¼ teaspoon freshly ground black pepper
2 medium tomatoes, chopped

Preheat the oven to 190°C/375°F/Gas Mark 5. Score the potatoes and bake for about 45 minutes, until tender. Measure the broccoli and beans into a steamer and steam until tender but still brightly coloured, about 12 minutes. Dissolve the yeast extract in the water and pour into a frying pan over a medium heat. When the liquid begins to bubble, sauté the onion until tender, 3–5 minutes, stirring often. Add the pepper and stir for 1 minute longer. Add the steamed broccoli and beans and the chopped tomato. Stir for 1 minute then cover the pan and remove from the heat. Slice the potatoes open and top with the bean and broccoli filling. Alternatively, scoop out the flesh, gently stir it into the broccoli mixture and spoon it all back into the potato skins. Serve at once.

Bean and Mushroom Cannelloni

Serves 4
Preparation time: 1 hour
✔ *LifePoints per serving: 53*
✘ *RiskPoints per serving: 2*

1 teaspoon yeast extract
60ml (2 fl oz) water
1 medium onion, finely chopped
225g (8oz) mushrooms, sliced
450g (1lb) cooked kidney beans, drained
½ teaspoon chilli powder or freshly ground black pepper
225g (8oz) (approximately 12) cannelloni
450g (1lb) spinach, washed and chopped
450g (1lb) tomatoes, sieved or chopped
3 cloves garlic, crushed
2 teaspoons dried oregano
chilli powder or black pepper, to taste
1 tablespoon fresh basil, finely chopped

Preheat the oven to 180°C/350°F/Gas Mark 4. Dissolve the yeast extract in the water and place in a saucepan over a medium heat. When the liquid begins to bubble, add the onions and stir for 3 minutes. Add the mushrooms, cover the pan and reduce the heat. Cook for 5 minutes then stir, cover the pan again and cook for a further 3 minutes. Add the kidney beans and the chilli and stir well, perhaps mashing the beans a little at the same time. Remove this mixture from the heat and use it to stuff the cannelloni.

Place the stuffed cannelloni in a casserole dish; any surplus filling may be placed around it in the dish. Pack the chopped spinach around the cannelloni. Mix the tomato, garlic, oregano and chilli together in a jug and pour over the cannelloni and spinach.

Cover the dish and bake for 20–25 minutes. Uncover it and return it to the oven for a further 10 minutes. Sprinkle the fresh basil over the dish and serve immediately.

Bean Pâté

Serves 8
Preparation time: 45 minutes, plus cooling and chilling time
✔ *LifePoints per serving: 11*
✘ *RiskPoints per serving: 0*

225g (8oz) dried red lentils, washed and drained
1 teaspoon yeast extract
570ml (1 pint) water
1 teaspoon turmeric
85g (3oz) rice flakes
1 teaspoon freshly ground black pepper or ½–1 teaspoon chilli powder
2 teaspoons ground ginger

Turn the lentils into a saucepan. Dissolve the yeast extract in the water, pour over the lentils, place on a medium – high flame and bring to a soft boil. Cover the pan, reduce the heat and simmer for 30 minutes, stirring occasionally. Add the turmeric, rice flakes, pepper and ginger and cook over a low flame for a further 5–10 minutes. Remove from the heat and spoon into a serving dish. Press the pâté well down into the dish. Allow to cool, then cover and chill before serving. This looks wonderful garnished with parsley or lemon slices.

Beans and Greens Salad

Serves 4
Preparation time: 35 minutes
✔ *LifePoints per serving: 33*
✘ *RiskPoints per serving: 2*

450g (1lb) broccoli, trimmed and cut into florets
2 medium carrots, shredded
3 spring onions, finely chopped
180g (6oz) chicory greens (escarole or batavia), chopped
450g (1lb) cooked or tinned kidney beans
juice of 1 lemon
½ teaspoon prepared mustard
¼–½ teaspoon freshly ground black pepper
salt to taste

Steam the broccoli for 10–12 minutes, until just tender but still bright green. Lift out of the steamer immediately and cool. Mix the carrots, onions, greens and cooled broccoli together in a large salad bowl. Drain the beans but reserve the final, thick broth. Add the beans to the salad. Mix the broth with the lemon juice, mustard and pepper. Add salt to taste and pour this over the salad. Toss and serve. This is a robust salad, filling on its own or over a baked potato or bowl of cold rice.

Beefless Stroganoff

Serves 4
Preparation time: 45 minutes
✔ *LifePoints per serving: 41*
✘ *RiskPoints per serving: 2*

1 teaspoon yeast extract
60ml (2fl oz) water
5–7 cloves garlic, finely chopped
1 large onion, finely chopped
225g (8oz) mushrooms, halved
100g (4oz) TVP chunks
2 tablespoons paprika
1 teaspoon cayenne
450g (1lb) chestnut purée
1 litre (2 pints) water
1 large green pepper, deseeded and diced

Dissolve the yeast extract in the water and place in a large saucepan over a medium heat. When the liquid bubbles, add the garlic and onion and sauté for 3–5 minutes, stirring constantly.

Add the mushrooms and cover the pan. Reduce the heat and cook for 7 minutes, stirring once in that time. Then stir in the TVP chunks to absorb all the liquid. Add the paprika, cayenne, chestnut purée and water and stir well. Bring to a low boil, cover the pan and reduce the heat. Leave to simmer gently for 20 minutes, stirring occasionally. Remove from the heat, stir in the green pepper and serve hot over rice.

Cabbage and Arame Salad

Serves 4
Preparation time: 30 minutes, plus standing time
✔ *LifePoints per serving: 6*
✗ *RiskPoints per serving: 0*

25g (1oz) arame seaweed
¼ white cabbage, finely shredded
2 medium carrots, shredded
3–5 spring onions, finely chopped or 1 small sweet onion, finely chopped
½ teaspoon freshly ground black pepper
juice of 1 lemon
2 tablespoons vinegar
2 teaspoons soy sauce

Rinse the arame under running water, then soak it in fresh cold water for 20 minutes. Lift it from the water, place it in a deep saucepan and cover with fresh water. Bring to a boil over a medium heat then reduce the heat and simmer, uncovered, for 15 minutes. Stir occasionally. Drain and put to one side.

Put the remaining ingredients in a large salad bowl, add the arame and mix well. Leave the salad to stand for 1 hour, or longer if desired, stirring once or twice during that time. Serve on a bed of chicory, radicchio or dandelion leaves (or any strong, slightly bitter leaf). A baked potato is an excellent accompaniment.

Carrot, Lentil and Ginger Salad

Serves 4
Preparation time: 1 hour
✔ *LifePoints per serving: 48*
✘ *RiskPoints per serving: 0*

100g (4oz) continental (brown) lentils
½ teaspoon freshly ground black pepper
juice of 1 lemon
450g (1lb) carrots, peeled and sliced julienne
1 teaspoon yeast extract
60ml (2fl oz) water
1 small onion, finely chopped
2 tablespoons fresh ginger, grated
100g (4oz) mushrooms, cleaned and quartered or sliced
½ bunch fresh coriander, chopped

Prepare the lentils first: wash them really well in cold water. Drain and cover in hot water. Leave for 5 minutes then drain and rub the lentils quite roughly to remove their skins. Cover in cold water and skim off the skins. You can repeat this procedure once or twice more if you like. Drain and turn into a pot, cover with fresh water and bring to the boil. Reduce the heat, partly cover the pan and simmer for 20–30 minutes, until the lentils are tender. Drain and stir in the black pepper and the lemon juice. Leave to cool in a large salad bowl.

Prepare the carrots: 'sliced julienne' means to slice into matchstick-size pieces, or as close to that as you can. Dissolve the yeast extract in the water and place in a saucepan over a medium heat. When the liquid begins to bubble, sauté the onion until clear and tender, about 3 minutes. Add the carrots, reduce the heat and cover the pan. Cook gently for about 7 minutes, stirring twice during that period. Use a little more water if necessary to prevent sticking. Add the ginger and stir for 1 minute. Add the mushrooms, cover the pan again and leave for 3–5 minutes, stirring once. Turn this mixture into the salad bowl with the lentils and leave to cool. When quite cool add the chopped coriander and stir well. Serve at once or chill in the refrigerator until ready to serve.

Celery and Barley Soup

Serves 4
Preparation time: 1 hour 15 minutes
✔ *LifePoints per serving: 27*
✘ *RiskPoints per serving: 1*

2 teaspoons yeast extract
60ml (2 fl oz) water
3 cloves garlic, finely chopped
1 medium onion, finely chopped
1 teaspoon freshly ground black pepper
4 stalks celery, thinly sliced
1 teaspoon dried marjoram
1 teaspoon turmeric
55g (2oz) barley
2 bay leaves
1.5 litres (3 pints) water
450g (1lb) green beans, trimmed and sliced
450g (1lb) broccoli, cut into florets

Dissolve the yeast extract in the water and pour into a large saucepan over a medium heat. When the liquid bubbles, sauté the garlic and onion until tender, about 3 minutes. Add the pepper and celery and continue to sauté for a further 5–7 minutes, stirring often. Cover the pan during this time if you wish and reduce the heat or add a tiny bit of water if the sauté is too brisk. When the celery is tender, stir in the marjoram and turmeric. Add the barley, bay and water and bring to the boil. Cover the pan, reduce the heat and simmer for 30 minutes. Add the beans and broccoli and simmer for a further 15 minutes. Adjust the seasoning and serve.

Cock-a-Leekie

Serves 6
Preparation time: 1 hour 15 minutes
✔ *LifePoints per serving: 38*
✘ *RiskPoints per serving: 3*

225g (8oz) TVP chunks, chicken flavour
100g (4oz) barley
4 large leeks, thinly sliced
4 stalks celery, thinly sliced
2 teaspoons freshly ground black pepper
2 bay leaves
1 teaspoon fresh thyme
2 teaspoons yeast extract
2 litres (4 pints) water

Measure the TVP into a large saucepan and pour the barley round it. Arrange the leeks and celery over this and sprinkle with the pepper. Add the bay leaves and thyme. Dilute the yeast extract in the water and pour over all. Cover the pan and place over a medium heat. Bring to the boil, stir, then reduce the heat, cover the pan again and leave to simmer very gently for at least 1 hour. Stir once or twice during this time. When the barley and TVP are very tender, serve hot with more freshly ground black pepper.

Cream of Mushroom Soup

Serves 4
Preparation time: 35 minutes
✔ *LifePoints per serving: 16*
✘ *RiskPoints per serving: 13*

This soup compares rather well with its traditional parent: cream of mushroom soup usually rates 8 LifePoints and 59 RiskPoints per serving.

450g (1lb) mushrooms, cleaned and finely chopped
juice of 1 lemon
1 tablespoon oil
1 small onion, finely chopped
1 teaspoon yeast extract
½ teaspoon freshly ground black pepper
¼ teaspoon ground nutmeg
1 tablespoon plain flour
425ml (¾ pint) soya milk
570ml (1 pint) water or vegetable stock
2 spring onions, finely chopped

Prepare the mushrooms and turn them into a bowl. Pour the lemon juice over them, stir well and leave to stand while you prepare the soup. Heat the oil in a large saucepan over a medium heat. Add the onion and sauté until it is clear and tender, about 3 minutes. Add the yeast extract, pepper and nutmeg and stir for 1 further minute. Sprinkle the flour over the sauté and stir to make a thick paste, or roux. Blend the milk and water together and add to the roux, a little at a time, stirring after each addition. Mix in the mushrooms and their juices and stir well. Leave over a low heat, stirring occasionally, for 7–10 minutes. Add more liquid if you wish. Serve hot with a garnish of chopped spring onions.

Creamed Vegetable Soup

Serves 4
Preparation time: 45 minutes
✔ *LifePoints per serving: 38*
✘ *RiskPoints per serving: 1*

100g (4oz) red lentils, washed and drained
1 teaspoon freshly ground black pepper
1 whole cauliflower, finely chopped, including good outer leaves
2 medium carrots, peeled and diced
450g (1lb) broccoli, trimmed and chopped
1 bulb garlic, peeled
2 teaspoons yeast extract
1.25 litres (2½ pints) water
2 tablespoons fresh parsley, finely chopped

Put the lentils and pepper into a large saucepan. Add the chopped vegetables and stir well. Dissolve the yeast extract in 285ml (½ pint) of the water and pour onto the vegetables. Cover the pan and place over a low heat for 15 minutes. Stir, add the remaining water and place over a medium heat. Simmer for 10–15 minutes, until the vegetables are just tender and the lentils are completely cooked. Turn the whole mixture through a mouli or hand blender, return it to the pan and bring back to a simmer. Add more water as you like. Serve the soup and garnish each serving with fresh parsley.

Fried Vegetable Cake

Serves 2
Preparation time: 45 minutes
✔ *LifePoints per serving: 27*
✘ *RiskPoints per serving: 1*

2 teaspoons yeast extract
140ml (¼ pint) water
1 small onion, finely chopped
1 large potato, grated
1 medium carrot, grated
150g (5oz) (approximately) broccoli, finely chopped
½ teaspoon freshly ground black pepper

Dissolve the yeast extract in the water and pour half into a large frying pan. Place over a medium heat; when the liquid begins to bubble sauté the onion for 2–3 minutes, stirring often. Mix the remaining ingredients together in a mixing bowl and add this mixture to the sauté. Stir for 1–2 minutes, then spread the mixture evenly in the pan, cover, reduce the heat and leave to cook for 5 minutes. Slice the cake into halves or quarters with a spatula; lift each section and turn it over. Add the remaining yeast extract mixture as you do so. Cover the pan and cook for 5 minutes. Uncover and test that the vegetables are tender. Lift from the pan and serve hot or cold with salad or steamed greens.

Fruit and Cereal Snack Bars

Serves 6
Preparation time: 45 minutes
✔ *LifePoints per serving: 40*
✘ *RiskPoints per serving: 13*

225g (8oz) plain flour
100g (4oz) wheat germ
55g (2oz) Grape Nuts cereal
2 teaspoons baking powder
2 teaspoons ground ginger
1 teaspoon ground allspice

1 teaspoon ground cinnamon
1 teaspoon ground nutmeg
100g (4oz) dates, finely chopped
100g (4oz) currants
55g (2oz) mixed peel
2 tablespoons tahini
4 tablespoons blackstrap molasses
570ml (1 pint) hot water

Preheat the oven to 180°C/350°F/Gas Mark 4 and lightly oil a
23 × 33cm (9 × 13 inch) cake tin. Mix all the dry ingredients and
the fruits together in a large mixing bowl. Stir the tahini, molasses
and hot water together in a jug, until the molasses has dissolved.
Pour this mixture over the dry mix, stir well and turn the batter
into the tin. Bake for 30 minutes, until a toothpick inserted comes
out clean. Cool on a wire rack, then slice and serve.

Garden Fresh Dip

Serves 4
Preparation time: 20 minutes, including steaming
✔ LifePoints per serving: 9
✘ RiskPoints per serving: 4

225g (8oz) fresh garden peas, steamed
225g (8oz) plain soya yogurt
1 tablespoon fresh mint, finely chopped
salt to taste

Put all the ingredients into a bowl and mash them together with a
fork. For a smoother texture, use a blender.

Garlic Bread

Serves 4
Preparation time: 30 minutes
✔ LifePoints per serving: 12
✘ RiskPoints per serving: 4

2 whole bulbs of garlic
25g (1oz) fresh parsley, finely chopped

1 teaspoon yeast extract
2 baguettes

Preheat the oven to 180°C/350°F/Gas Mark 4. Separate the bulbs of garlic into cloves and discard the surplus skin, though keeping each clove covered in its own skin. Drop the cloves into a pan of boiling water and boil for 5–7 minutes, depending on their size. Lift the cloves from the water and cool until hand-hot. Peel the cloves and turn the soft flesh into a bowl. When all the cloves have been peeled, mash the flesh, adding the parsley and yeast extract to make a paste. Slice the baguettes in half along their length and spread each half with some of the garlic mixture. Close the baguettes and wrap in kitchen foil. Bake for 12 minutes and serve warm, one half baguette for each serving.

NOTE: Of course, the bread may be whatever sort you like, sliced in whatever manner you like. Also, the parsley may be omitted or replaced by another fresh herb such as basil or thyme.

Green Garden Sandwiches

Serves 4
Preparation time: 30 minutes, including time to steam the asparagus and make the Dip
✔ *LifePoints per serving: 23*
✘ *RiskPoints per serving: 8*

8 thin slices wholewheat bread
1 x recipe Garden Fresh Dip (see page 128)
225g (8oz) asparagus, steamed and cooled
1 bunch watercress, finely chopped
4 leaves cos lettuce

Spread the bread slices lavishly with the Dip. Arrange the steamed asparagus spears over the dip, sprinkle with lots of watercress and top with lettuce. Close the sandwich, slice and serve.

Heart of Gold Roasted Pumpkin

Serves 4
Preparation time: 55 minutes
✔ *LifePoints per serving: 10*
✘ *RiskPoints per serving: 0*

1 small pumpkin or squash (approximately 900g (2lb))
1 teaspoon yeast extract
60ml (2fl oz) water
1 medium onion, thinly sliced
½ teaspoon freshly ground black pepper
4 tablespoons fresh parsley, finely chopped
½ teaspoon ground cinnamon

Prepare the pumpkin: quarter it and remove the seed pulp; discard the seeds or grow them in your garden. Rinse the pumpkin quarters and score their flesh on the inside of the curve only.

Preheat the oven to 180°C/350°F/Gas Mark 4. Dissolve the yeast extract in the water and place in a frying pan over a medium heat. When the liquid begins to bubble, add the onion slices, carefully breaking the slices apart as you do so. Sauté the onion for 3 minutes, until it begins to get tender. Remove from the heat.

Mix the pepper, parsley and cinnamon together in a small bowl. Take one-quarter of this mixture and rub it into the scored area of a piece of pumpkin. Repeat for each piece until all the mixture is used. Now place the pumpkin quarters in a roasting tray in which there is about ½ inch of water. Lay some of the sautéed onion slices onto each piece of pumpkin and bake for 25–30 minutes. Test the pumpkin is cooked by piercing the flesh with a fork. Serve hot alongside rice and steamed greens.

Hearty Goulash

Serves 4
Preparation time: 45 minutes
✔ *LifePoints per serving: 42*
✘ *RiskPoints per serving: 5*

1 teaspoon yeast extract
60ml (2fl oz) water
5–7 cloves garlic, finely chopped
1 medium onion, finely chopped
1 teaspoon freshly ground black pepper
½ teaspoon chilli powder
1 × 125g (4½oz) packet sun-dried tomatoes, quartered
100g (4oz) TVP chunks
570–850ml (1–1½ pint) water
140g (5oz) tomato paste
450g (1lb) potatoes, peeled and quartered
1 tablespoon paprika
2 tablespoons apricot jam

Dissolve the yeast extract in the water and place in a large saucepan over a medium heat. When the liquid bubbles, add the garlic and onion and sauté for 3–5 minutes, stirring constantly. Add the pepper and chilli powder and stir for 1 minute, then add the sun-dried tomatoes and stir for a further minute. Add the TVP chunks and the water and bring to a low boil. Stir in the tomato paste and the potatoes, cover the pan and simmer gently for about 20 minutes; add more water if necessary. Add the paprika and apricot jam and stir well. Remove from the heat and serve immediately or leave to stand 2–4 hours, then reheat. Serve over rice, buckwheat or on its own in a big soup bowl.

Lasagne Bolognaise

Serves 4
Preparation time: 1 hour, plus optional standing time
✔ *LifePoints per serving: 61*
✘ *RiskPoints per serving: 10*

1 teaspoon yeast extract
60ml (2fl oz) water
7 cloves garlic, finely chopped
1 medium onion, finely chopped
1 teaspoon freshly ground black pepper
100g (4oz) TVP mince
1 × 400g (14oz) tin chopped tomatoes

285g (10oz) tomato paste
570ml (1 pint) water
1 teaspoon dried oregano
2 tablespoons fresh parsley, finely chopped
1 tablespoon fresh basil, finely chopped
450g (1lb) lasagne noodles
450g (1lb) chicory greens (escarole or batavia), washed and
chopped
55g (2oz) breadcrumbs
½ teaspoon freshly ground black pepper
2 tablespoons fresh parsley, finely chopped
1 tablespoon fresh basil, finely chopped

Dissolve the yeast extract in the water and place in a saucepan
over a medium heat. When the liquid begins to bubble, sauté the
garlic for 2 minutes. Add the onion and sauté for a further 3
minutes, stirring often. Mix in the pepper, stir well and then add
the mince. Add the chopped tomatoes, paste, water and oregano
and bring to a simmer, stirring well. Adjust the liquid if necessary
to make a thick, slightly gloopy mixture. Stir in the fresh herbs,
cover the pan and remove from the heat. You may continue the
preparations immediately or put the sauce aside for up to 4
hours.

Parboil the lasagne in a large pan of salted, boiling water for
about 4 minutes. Preheat the oven to 180°C/350°F/Gas Mark 4.
Pour a ladleful of sauce into a casserole and arrange lasagne over
it. Sprinkle some of the chopped greens over the lasagne and
cover with another layer of sauce. Continue in this way – layering
sauce, lasagne, greens – until all the ingredients are used, ending
with a topping of sauce.

Mix the breadcrumbs with the pepper and herbs and sprinkle
over the top layer of sauce. Bake for 40 minutes. Leave to stand
for 5 minutes, then slice and serve hot.

Marinated Steak and Mushrooms with Roast Potatoes

Serves 4
Preparation time: 1 hour, plus marinating time
✔ *LifePoints per serving: 65*
✘ *RiskPoints per serving: 4*

for the steak:
225g (8oz) TVP chunks
225g (8oz) button mushrooms, cleaned and trimmed
140ml (¼ pint) cider vinegar
2 tablespoons soy sauce
180ml (6 fl oz) red wine
6 whole cloves
12 whole peppercorns
1 3-inch piece cinnamon
25g (1 oz) fresh ginger, thinly sliced
6 cloves garlic, finely chopped
1 small onion, finely chopped
570ml–1 litre (1–2 pints) apple juice
2 teaspoons arrowroot (kuzu)

for the potatoes:
900g (2lb) potatoes, scrubbed and quartered
2 teaspoons yeast extract
140ml (¼ pint) water
2 teaspoons dried rosemary
1 teaspoon freshly ground black pepper

Measure the TVP and the mushrooms into a large mixing bowl and stir gently. Blend the vinegar, soy sauce, wine, spices, ginger, garlic and onion together in a jug. Add 570ml (1 pint) of the apple juice and pour this mixture over the steak and mushrooms. Leave to marinate for at least 1 hour, but ideally 4–6 hours or all day. Stir once or twice during this time and add more apple juice if necessary to ensure the TVP fully rehydrates.

Turn this mixture into a saucepan, removing the cloves, peppercorns and cinnamon if you wish, and bring to a boil over a medium heat. Reduce the heat, cover the pan and simmer gently for 20–30 minutes, until the steak is very tender. Again, add more apple juice if necessary.

Meanwhile, preheat the oven to 180°C/350°F/Gas Mark 4.

Prepare the potatoes: dip each quarter in the yeast extract dissolved in the water. Arrange on a baking tray and pour the remaining yeast extract mixture over them. Sprinkle the rosemary and pepper over, cover the tray with kitchen foil and bake for 30 minutes. Remove the foil and bake for a further 10 minutes, basting with a little more diluted yeast extract if necessary.

Just before serving, dissolve the arrowroot in 1–2 tablespoons apple juice or water and stir this into the simmering steak and mushroom mixture. Cook for a further 5 minutes while the sauce thickens. Arrange the roasted potatoes in a ring on each plate and ladle some of the steak and mushrooms into the centre. Serve hot, with greens and steamed carrots around the outer edge of the plate.

Melon and Apricot Smoothie

Serves 2
Preparation time: 45 minutes
✔ *LifePoints per serving: 27*
✘ *RiskPoints per serving: 2*

100g (4oz) dehydrated apricots
285ml (½ pint) orange juice
1 ripe canteloupe melon
2 bananas
some ice cubes, optional

Wash the apricots and chop them finely. Pour the orange juice over and soak them for at least 2 hours, though all day or overnight is fine too. Turn the apricots and juice into a food processor (or into a deep bowl if you are using a hand-held blender). Halve the melon, remove the seeds and scoop the flesh into the blender. Peel the bananas and add to the rest of the fruit in the blender. If you wish, add the ice cubes as well, then purée the mixture and pour immediately into tall glasses and serve.

New Pastry

Serves 6 – makes sufficient for one 30.5cm (12 inch) flan
Preparation time: 35 minutes
✔ *LifePoints per serving: 28*
✘ *RiskPoints per serving: 5*

285g (10oz) Grape Nuts breakfast cereal
100g (4oz) oat flakes

2 teaspoons spice, to taste (i.e. freshly ground black pepper for a savoury flan; spices such as cinnamon, nutmeg, cloves or allspice for a sweet flan)
200ml (7fl oz) water

Blend the dry ingredients together in a bowl. Add the liquid, stir well and leave to stand for 10 minutes, stirring once or twice during that time. Turn the mixture into a non-stick or lightly oiled flan or pie dish and press into place. Bake blind for 20 minutes in a hot oven or fill and bake as per your chosen recipe.

This pastry works well for a raised pie: simply reserve about a quarter of the mixture and press the remaining pastry into place in a deep pie dish. Lightly flour a board and roll the reserved pastry to fit the pie dish. Lift very carefully onto the filled pie, press the edges together and bake.

Onion and Fennel Flan

Serves 6
Preparation time: 1 hour 15 minutes
✔ *LifePoints per serving: 38*
✘ *RiskPoints per serving: 11*

1 x recipe for New Pastry (see page 134)
½ bulb fresh fennel, finely chopped
1 large onion, thinly sliced
225g (8oz) broccoli, trimmed and cut into florets
1 teaspoon paprika
285g (10oz) silken tofu, drained
140ml (¼ pint) soya milk

Preheat the oven to 180°C/350°F/Gas Mark 4. Prepare the pastry and press it into a large (30cm/12 inch) flan dish. Arrange the chopped fennel in the flan case and the onion slices over the fennel. Place the broccoli florets, stalk-side-down if possible, evenly over the onion and sprinkle the paprika over all. Whisk the tofu and soya milk together and pour over the vegetables. Bake for 40 minutes. Cool for 5 minutes on a wire rack, then slice and serve.

Pineapple Glazed Apples and Oranges Bake

Serves 4
Preparation time: 45 minutes
✔ LifePoints per serving: 21
✘ RiskPoints per serving: 3

2 tablespoons brown sugar
4 rings of pineapple
4 apples, peeled, cored and quartered
2 oranges, peeled and segmented, retain zest
55g (2oz) Grape Nuts
55g (2oz) oat flakes
1 teaspoon ground cinnamon
1 teaspoon ground cloves
120ml (4 fl oz) pineapple juice

Preheat the oven to 180°C/350°F/Gas Mark 4. This dish may be prepared in a single baking dish or in four individual ramekins. Sprinkle the brown sugar over the bottom of the dish. Arrange the pineapple rings on top and place the apple quarters carefully over the rings. Chop the orange segments and sprinkle over the apples. Mix the Grape Nuts, orange zest, oats and spices together in a bowl and spread this mixture over the fruits. Drizzle the pineapple juice over the dry mix. Bake for 30 minutes. Serve hot.

Polenta with Black Bean and Mushroom Sauce

Serves 4
Preparation time: 1 hour 15 minutes, plus soaking time
✔ LifePoints per serving: 27
✘ RiskPoints per serving: 4

570ml (1 pint) water
100g (4oz) coarse cornmeal
225g (8oz) black beans (i.e. turtle), soaked and drained
1 large onion, finely chopped
1 bulb garlic, coarsely chopped
2 tablespoons fresh ginger, grated
2 teaspoons freshly ground black pepper

1 teaspoon yeast extract
60ml (2 fl oz) water
225g (8oz) mushrooms, cleaned and halved or quartered
2 fresh tomatoes, chopped

Bring the water to the boil in a saucepan and pour the cornmeal into it, stirring all the while. Simmer for 20–30 minutes over a low–medium heat to make polenta. Pour into a non-stick tray or flan dish and leave to cool.

Soak the beans all day or overnight then drain them, rinse and turn them into a pressure cooker and just cover with fresh water. Cook at pressure for 20 minutes.

Turn the beans immediately into a large pan and add the onion, garlic, ginger and pepper. Place over a medium heat and simmer for 15 minutes. Remove from the heat. Dissolve the yeast extract in the water and pour into a saucepan over a medium heat. When the liquid begins to bubble, add the mushrooms, stir well and cover the pan. Reduce the heat and leave them to cook for 3–5 minutes. Stir, cover the pan again and leave to cook for a final 3–5 minutes. The mushrooms should release their juices and become aromatic. Stir the mushrooms and their juices into the cooked beans; add the chopped tomato and stir well.

Slice the cooled polenta into four pieces and lift each of these onto a plate. Ladle the beans over the polenta and serve with steamed greens.

NOTE: the polenta may be served hot, if preferred, in its more liquid state. In this case, make it while the sauce cooks and spoon it immediately into a bowl with the beans.

Pourgouri Salad

Serves 4
Preparation time: 35 minutes, plus cooling time
✔ *LifePoints per serving: 22*
✗ *RiskPoints per serving: 1*

1 teaspoon yeast extract
570ml (1 pint) boiling water
225g (8oz) pourgouri (i.e. cracked wheat, bulghur)

½ teaspoon freshly ground black pepper
225g (8oz) spinach, cleaned and chopped
3 spring onions, finely chopped
1 small red pepper, finely chopped
1 tablespoon fresh parsley, finely chopped
3 tablespoons fresh coriander, finely chopped

Dissolve the yeast extract in the boiling water and return to the boil. Add the remaining ingredients, stir well, cover the pan and remove from the heat. Leave to stand for about 20 minutes then stir and cover the pan again. Allow to cool completely before serving. This salad may be chilled. It is excellent with a little orange or lemon juice drizzled over it and makes a wonderful filling for pitta.

Quiche Alsace

Serves 6
Preparation time: 1 hour 15 minutes
✔ LifePoints per serving: 39
✘ RiskPoints per serving: 5

1 × recipe for New Pastry (see page 134)
3 medium potatoes, scrubbed and thinly sliced
1 large onion, thinly sliced
¼ red cabbage, shredded
100g (4oz) sweet chestnuts, steamed and mashed
2 teaspoons freshly ground black pepper
2 teaspoons dried sage
2 teaspoons yeast extract
140ml (¼ pint) water

Preheat the oven to 180°C/350°F/Gas Mark 4. Press the pastry into a deep pie dish and arrange a layer of potato slices over it. Place a layer of onion, then cabbage, then chestnut over the potatoes, using half of each of these three foods. Mix the pepper and sage together and sprinkle half of this mixture over the chestnuts. Place a thin layer of potato slices over the herbs. Now use the remaining ingredients and layer in this order: onions, cabbage, chestnut and potato. Sprinkle the remaining pepper and herb mixture over all. Dissolve the yeast extract in the water and pour this evenly over the pie. Cover with kitchen foil and bake for 30 minutes. Remove the foil and bake for a further 10–15 minutes. Serve hot.

Raspberry Trifle

Serves 4
Preparation time: 40 minutes, plus chilling time
✔ *LifePoints per serving: 23*
✘ *RiskPoints per serving: 9*

8 large shreds-of-wheat breakfast cereal biscuits
340g (12oz) plain yogurt
900g (2lbs) lemon sorbet
900g (2lbs) fresh raspberries, washed and drained

Slice the biscuits in half along their length, reserving any crumbs. Use about half the biscuit halves to line a large ramekin or pudding basin. Spoon half of the yogurt into the dish, spreading it all around to cover the biscuits. Use just under half the sorbet in the same manner, spreading it over the whole of the inner surface if possible. Add one third of the raspberries and place a layer of biscuit halves over them. Spread a dollop of yogurt over the biscuits, then more sorbet and another one third of the berries. Repeat this sequence once more: biscuits, yogurt, sorbet, berries. Top with any remaining sorbet and yogurt and finally with biscuits or crumbs of biscuits. Carefully press the top of the trifle firmly down with a saucer or the back of a large spoon. Chill in the freezer for 30–60 minutes then keep in the refrigerator until ready to serve.

Red-Hot Vegetable Curry

Serves 4
Preparation time: 45 minutes
✔ *LifePoints per serving: 49*
✘ *RiskPoints per serving: 1*

2 teaspoons yeast extract
140ml (¼ pint) water

1 whole bulb garlic, finely chopped
1 large onion, finely chopped
450g (1lb) carrots, peeled and chopped
450g (1lb) parsnips, peeled and cubed
450g (1lb) spinach, washed, drained and chopped
1½ teaspoons cumin
1 teaspoon mustard seeds
½ teaspoon chilli powder
4 cardamom pods, slightly crushed
1 teaspoon turmeric
juice of 1 lemon

Dissolve the yeast extract in the water and pour half of this mixture into a large saucepan over a medium heat. When the liquid begins to bubble, add half the chopped garlic and all of the onion and sauté for 3–5 minutes, stirring often. Add the vegetables, stir well and reduce the heat. Cover the pan and leave to cook for about 20 minutes over a low heat, stirring occasionally. If the vegetables begin to stick, add just enough water to cover the bottom of the pan. (NOTE: this is a 'dry' curry, with little sauce except the juices from the vegetables. Should you want more liquid, simply add more water.)

Heat the remaining yeast extract mixture in a small pan and sauté the remaining garlic in it, about 2 minutes. Add the cumin and mustard seeds and stir for 1 minute. Add the chilli, cardamom and turmeric, stir well and remove from the heat. Stir this sauté into the cooked vegetables and drizzle the lemon juice over all. Serve with rice.

Refreshing Pasta Salad

Serves 4
Preparation time: 35 minutes
✔ *LifePoints per serving: 23*
✘ *RiskPoints per serving: 6*

100g (4oz) pasta shapes (i.e. spirals, shells, bows)
225g (8oz) cooked chick peas, drained
zest and juice of 2 lemons
¼ teaspoon freshly ground black pepper

3 spring onions, finely chopped
1 green pepper, finely chopped
225g (8oz) fresh, raw peas
2 medium tomatoes, chopped
25g (1oz) fresh parsley, finely chopped
1 tablespoon fresh mint, finely chopped

Bring a large pot of salted water to the boil and add the pasta. Stir well and leave to simmer for about 12 minutes. Meanwhile, measure the chick peas into a large salad bowl and pour the lemon juice and zest over them. Sprinkle with the black pepper, onions, green pepper, peas and tomatoes. Add the herbs, stir well and leave to stand. When the pasta has cooked, drain and cool it under running water. Drain again and add to the salad. Stir well and serve immediately, though this will keep in the refrigerator for one day.

Sloppy Joes

Serves 4
Preparation time: 35 minutes
✔ *LifePoints per serving: 37*
✘ *RiskPoints per serving: 4*

1 teaspoon yeast extract
60ml (2 fl oz) water
7 cloves garlic, finely chopped
1 medium onion, finely chopped
½ teaspoon chilli powder
1 small chilli, finely chopped (optional)
100g (4oz) TVP mince
1 × 400g (14oz) tin chopped tomatoes
285g (10oz) tomato paste
140ml (¼ pint) apple juice
4 tablespoons fresh parsley, finely chopped
2 tablespoons fresh basil, finely chopped

Dissolve the yeast extract in the water and place in a saucepan over a medium heat. When the liquid begins to bubble, add the garlic and onion and sauté for 3–5 minutes, stirring often. Add the chilli powder, chilli and TVP mince and stir for 1 minute. Mix in the tomatoes, paste and apple juice and simmer gently for 20 minutes. Add the herbs, remove from the heat and serve immediately.

Sloppy Joes are traditionally served over a toasted bun – similar to beans on toast – but you may serve it over rice or millet.

Spiced Garden Beans

Serves 4
Preparation time: 25 minutes, plus chilling time
✔ *LifePoints per serving: 45*
✘ *RiskPoints per serving: 3*

450g (1lb) fresh broad beans, cleaned
450g (1lb) green beans, cleaned and sliced
1 small onion, very thinly sliced
90ml (3 fl oz) cider or raspberry vinegar
½ teaspoon freshly ground black pepper
2 teaspoons fresh ginger, grated
zest of 1 lemon

Steam or boil the beans until they are just tender, about 12 minutes. Have the onion ready and immediately the beans are cooked, drain them and turn them into a large bowl with the onion. Stir well. Mix the remaining ingredients together and pour over the beans and onion. Leave aside to cool, stirring occasionally, and chill in the refrigerator if desired. This is excellent beside the Wild Rice Risotto (page 146).

Spiced Kidney Bean Ragoût

Serves 4
Preparation time: 45 minutes, plus soaking overnight
✘ *RiskPoints per serving: 1*
✔ *LifePoints per serving: 19*

225g (8oz) kidney beans, washed and drained
1 teaspoon yeast extract
60ml (2 fl oz) water

1 medium onion, finely chopped
1 red pepper, thinly sliced and chopped
2 tablespoons fresh ginger, grated
1 fresh chilli, finely chopped
½ teaspoon chilli powder
½ bunch fresh coriander, finely chopped
340ml (12 fl oz) tomato juice

Soak the beans overnight or all day. Drain them, rinse and turn into a pressure cooker and just cover with fresh water. Cook at pressure for 20–25 minutes. Drain, retaining the thick juices, and turn into a large saucepan and place over a low heat.

Meanwhile, dissolve the yeast extract in the water and place in a frying pan over a medium heat. When the liquid begins to bubble, add the onion and red pepper and sauté for 5–7 minutes, stirring often. Add the ginger, chilli and coriander and stir for 1 minute. Pour the tomato juice over and bring to the boil.

Pour this sauce over the hot beans and simmer for 5–10 minutes. Serve immediately with rice or corn bread. For a more intense spiciness, leave the beans to stand for up to 4 hours then reheat.

Spicy Foule Medames

Serves 4
Preparation time: 3 hours, plus soaking overnight
✔ *LifePoints per serving: 29*
✘ *RiskPoints per serving: 2*

450g (1lb) foule medames or black beans, washed and soaked overnight
2 teaspoons yeast extract
90ml (3 fl oz) water
2 teaspoons freshly ground black pepper
1 teaspoon ground allspice
½ teaspoon ground cloves
7 whole cloves
3 bay leaves
7 cardamom, bruised

1 whole bulb garlic, coarsely chopped or 3 tablespoons dried garlic flakes
55g (2oz) fresh ginger, peeled and thinly sliced
1.5 litres (3 pints) vegetable stock

Drain the soaked beans and rinse them well. Drain again. Dissolve the yeast extract in the water and place in a large saucepan over a medium heat. When the liquid bubbles, add all the spices, garlic and ginger and stir for about 3 minutes. Add the drained beans and the vegetable stock and bring to the boil. Cover the pan, reduce the heat and simmer gently for about 3 hours, until the beans are very tender (they should crush easily when pressed against the roof of the mouth with the tongue). Stir occasionally during this time. Serve hot or cold, over steamed rice or millet, over a baked potato or in a bowl all by itself.

Stuffed Cabbage Leaves in Rosemary Sauce

Serves 4
Preparation time: 1 hour
✔ *LifePoints per serving: 55*
✘ *RiskPoints per serving: 15*

8 leaves Chinese or white cabbage

for the filling:
450g (1lb) spinach, chopped
450g (1lb) potatoes, peeled and steamed
1 teaspoon yeast extract
60ml (2fl oz) water
6 cloves garlic
1½ teaspoon fresh rosemary, finely chopped
½ teaspoon fresh thyme, finely chopped
55g (2oz) wheat germ
4 tomatoes, finely chopped

for the sauce:
4 teaspoons fresh rosemary, finely chopped
285ml (½ pint) boiling water
1 tablespoon oil

1 small onion, finely chopped
1 teaspoon fresh rosemary, finely chopped
1 tablespoon plain flour
285ml (½ pint) soya milk

Blanch the cabbage leaves in boiling water for 60–90 seconds. Lift out and cool.

Mash the chopped spinach and potatoes together in a mixing bowl. Dissolve the yeast extract in the water and place in a small pan over a medium heat. When the liquid begins to bubble, add the garlic and sauté for about 3 minutes. Add the pepper, rosemary and thyme and stir for 1 minute. Stir this sauté into the mashed greens and potato, then add the wheat germ and chopped tomatoes. Stir briefly.

Place a spoonful of the filling mixture in the centre of a cabbage leaf and roll the leaf round it, folding in the edges as you do so. Place the stuffed leaf edge-side-down in a casserole and repeat until all the leaves are filled.

Measure the rosemary into a teapot and pour the boiling water over. Leave to steep for at least 10 minutes, then strain into a jug. Heat the oil in a saucepan and sauté the onion until clear and tender, about 3 minutes over a medium heat. Add the remaining rosemary, finely chopped, and stir for 1 minute longer. Sprinkle the flour over the sauté and stir to make a thick paste, or roux. Add the milk and rosemary tea, a little at a time, stirring after each addition to make a sauce.

Pour the sauce over the stuffed leaves, cover the casserole and bake for 20 minutes. Uncover and bake for a final 5 minutes. Serve hot with rice or millet and steamed pumpkin.

Sun-Dried Tomato Bolognaise

Serves 4
Preparation time: 25 minutes, plus 2 hours standing time
✔ *LifePoints per serving: 37*
✘ *RiskPoints per serving: 7*

1 teaspoon yeast extract
60ml (2 fl oz) water
3–5 cloves garlic, finely chopped

1 medium onion, finely chopped
1 teaspoon freshly ground black pepper
55g (2oz) TVP mince
285g (10oz) tomato paste
1 × 125g (4½oz) packet sun-dried tomatoes, finely chopped
570–850ml (1–1½ pints) water
2 tablespoons fresh parsley, finely chopped
1 tablespoon fresh basil, finely chopped
1 teaspoon soy sauce
½ teaspoon brown sugar
225g (8oz) pasta

Dissolve the yeast extract in the water and place in a saucepan over a medium heat. When the liquid begins to bubble, add the garlic and onion and sauté for 3–5 minutes, stirring often. Add the pepper and TVP and stir to absorb all the liquid. Add the remaining ingredients, except the pasta, stir well and simmer for 15 minutes over a low heat. Cover the pan, remove from the heat and leave to stand for at least 2 hours, if possible. You can serve it straightaway, but the flavour improves from standing.

Bring a large pan of salted water to the boil, add the pasta and simmer for 10–12 minutes. Drain and serve. Reheat the sauce and serve over the pasta. You could also use it as a sauce in lasagne or over rice.

Wild Rice Risotto

Serves 4
Preparation time: 45 minutes
✔ *LifePoints per serving: 22*
✘ *RiskPoints per serving: 3*

2 teaspoons yeast extract
140ml (¼ pint) water
6 cloves garlic, finely chopped
1 medium onion, finely chopped
1 teaspoon freshly ground black pepper
100g (4oz) wild rice, washed and drained
100g (4oz) brown rice, washed and drained

3 tablespoons tomato paste
140ml (¼ pint) water
425ml (¾ pint) water or vegetable stock
2 tablespoons fresh parsley
100g (4oz) fresh mung beansprouts

Dissolve the yeast extract in the water and place in a large saucepan over a medium heat. When the liquid begins to bubble, add the garlic and onion and stir for 3–5 minutes. Add the pepper and the rices and stir until all the liquid has been absorbed. Dissolve the tomato paste in the water and add this to the rice. Again, stir until all the liquid has been absorbed. Add the remaining liquid, cover the pan, reduce the heat and simmer until all the liquid has been absorbed and the rices are tender. (You may need to add a little more water, in which case boil it first, then add it.) When the rice is cooked, immediately stir in the parsley and beansprouts, cover the pan again and leave to stand for 5 minutes. Serve immediately, though this is excellent cold with a little orange zest grated over each serving.

PART FOUR: THE LIFEPOINTS LIFESTYLE

What happens after Day Seven of the Kick-Start? The rest of your life! Use the four to six weeks which follow to achieve some additional basic goals:

- Become very familiar with the LifePoints and RiskPoints listings.
- Use the experience of the Kick-Start and the tips which follow to develop two or three full-day menus which suit you very well.
- Practise one or two new cookery methods which help to improve your enjoyment of, and add LifePoints to, the food you eat.
- Exercise every day using the Kick-Start Stretches and the Walk One Mile set of guidelines.
- Gradually discover if there is another form of exercise you would also enjoy and begin to practise it.
- Continue to evaluate your health and fitness and to monitor your weight. Weigh yourself weekly for the first three months of the diet. At the end of four weeks, take the fat check test on page 25.
- Aim to rediscover your instinct for good food so that you can happily change your buying patterns as well as your cooking and eating patterns.

EAT YOUR LIFESTYLE!

First, eat food that is high in LifePoints and low in RiskPoints. That's easy enough now that you have an idea of what those foods are. In fact, it is likely that you won't need to refer to the LifePoints listings very often after another week or two; you will have rediscovered your own sense of what is good and bad food. There are some tips we can give you, however, on how to make the selection and preparation of good food easier. Use these to help design a diet that is truly yours: one that you enjoy, that fits into your lifestyle and that will keep you trim and in good health for the years ahead.

TIPS ON MENUS AND COOKING

When browsing through the recipes you will notice that we sauté without oil. Sautéing is a method which is very enticing as it produces those lovely aromas and sizzling sounds that start us all salivating with anticipation. How could we ever replace it? It took us a lot of tastings to discover the best alternative and we use it regularly in these recipes and in those in *The LifePoints Cookbook*.

We call it the **New Sauté** and it is very simple: Dissolve 1–2 teaspoons yeast extract in 60–90ml (2–3 fl oz) water and bring this to a quick simmer in a frying pan or saucepan over a medium heat. Add the onions, garlic or whatever is to be sautéed and stir for 2–5 minutes, or the recommended time. The aroma is enticing, the sizzle is there and the flavour and texture created is excellent. In addition, the yeast extract adds valuable LifePoints to your total.

Once you get familiar with the New Sauté, adjust it by trying other liquids, such as tomato sauce, in place of the yeast extract dilution.

Losing your taste for fatty foods is certainly something to look forward to but it doesn't mean that you will lose your taste for tasty foods! Now is your chance to explore more fully the world of herbs and spices as these, added at the right time and in the right quantities, will enrich the flavour and aroma of your meals.

● **Herbs,** if dried, are best added during cooking so that their essential oils distribute through the food. If fresh, they are often best added towards the end of cooking or just before serving so as not to lose the delicate flavours fresh herbs produce. For instance, fresh basil may be added to a tomato sauce almost as a garnish when you serve it, yet it will still impart that exquisite aroma and flavour to the whole dish. Experiment with your own cooking and even try growing a pot of basil, parsley or thyme on your windowsill or terrace so that you have these otherwise expensive condiments to hand.

● **Spices** are often best added at the sauté stage so that their essential oils distribute well but also 'mature' during the rest of the cooking process. Some spices, such as common or garden black pepper, are especially good added at this stage. Others, such as the curry collection of spices, are often best added just before the end of cooking so that their flavours do not deteriorate. Again, experiment, with a light hand to begin with, until you get to know the results you may expect.

● **Tea and coffee**   are, unfortunately, part of everyday life for most of us. However, you will notice that, in the Kick-Start, we listed only one cup in the daily menus. This is because most people take milk in their tea or coffee and milk means RiskPoints. If you can enjoy your drink without milk, then tea or coffee may be taken freely without adding RiskPoints to your diet. However, neither will add LifePoints and neither is likely to enhance your health. Perhaps now is a good opportunity to reduce your intake of these beverages and try, instead, the many herb teas and cereal coffees currently on the market. Both of us like strong flavours so we always choose a herb tea such as nettle or fennel and we enjoy a proper brew of yannoh, a strong Middle-Eastern cereal coffee.

There are many **fat-traps** waiting to add RiskPoints to your diet, sometimes without you noticing, as you can see from reading about tea and coffee. Whoever heard of fresh fruit without cream, for instance? And how can one have toasted crumpet without mopping an ooze of butter off the plate? Well, we know the power such traditional tastes and expectations have but we also know that within another few weeks your taste for fat will have diminished and you will, instead, look forward to the flavour of the food itself, without lashings of butter and cream disguising it. Here is a short list of **fat-trap avoidance** techniques:

● Toasted crumpets, bagels and bread are delicious with just yeast extract spread onto them. If you are not the extract sort, thinly sliced banana can be arranged onto the toast (or even spread a little bit) to give a rich, luscious bite. In fact, one of our favourites (we included it in a snack menu) is to mash sweet chestnuts with a little salt and pepper and spread this over a toast. Yummy!

● Fresh fruit is delicious with low-fat yogurt or a delicate **orange sauce** poured over it instead of the usual cream. Try this: dissolve 1 teaspoon arrowroot in 1 tablespoon cold water. Heat the juice of 1 orange to a simmer then stir in the arrowroot paste. Keep stirring over a medium–low heat while adding the juice of 1 or 2 more oranges, and their zest if you like. When the sauce has thickened, pour into a serving jug or bowl and drizzle a little over fresh fruit once it has cooled somewhat.

- Fresh fruit is also surprisingly good with a crispbread or ricecake crumbled over it, perhaps adding a pinch of ground cinnamon or allspice at the same time. As you will note from the listings, both of these crackers have zero RiskPoints.

- Tea and coffee are best served black, with lemon or not at all.

- An innocent sauté can easily use up to 90ml (3 fl oz) oil, without you ever *seeing* a drop of that oil again, except on your waistline. Please do try to use the New Sauté we describe on page 150.

- Baked potatoes love butter, right? Yes, but it just disappears into them and, like the sauté, you can easily eat several tablespoons of butter in a potato without really noticing. The same is true of mashed potatoes. If you really feel like having an extra flavour with your potato, use a tablespoon of one of the low-fat dressings (French, Italian and Thousand Island are all listed here). Meanwhile, enjoy the LifePoints gained by eating a baked spud with baked beans, coleslaw or your own spiced mixture of chopped pickle, green beans and chopped tomato.

- **Nuts** are fat traps! Avoid them during the first month or so of your diet, then add them with discretion. For instance, if you really must have something fatty on your toast, why not have tahini or one of the **nut-butters**? These at least have LifePoints and, by the way, usually a reduced number of RiskPoints per serving size as well. (Compare butter at 18 RiskPoints 0 LifePoints per 5g serving with tahini at 20 RiskPoints 5 LifePoints per 15g serving.) Similarly, a muesli that contains nuts has a much higher RiskPoints rating than a muesli that does not. Fortunately, nut-free mueslis are available from most supermarkets. Just in case, however, here is a *home-made muesli* that you can try. Amend it as you wish by adding high-LifePoints ingredients:

for 1 serving
25g (1oz) rolled oats
25g (1oz) wheat germ
25g (1oz) puffed rice

¼ teaspoon ground cinnamon
75g (2½oz) currants
1 fresh banana, sliced
¾ cup skimmed milk

✔ LifePoints 69
✘ RiskPoints 22

- Salads love a good dressing and these, usually, include fat. We applaud the availability of the many low-fat dressings now on the market and advise you to use these, with a light hand, instead.
- Similarly, steamed vegetables can sometimes seem to cry out for a dab of butter, just like granny used to serve them. We have lost the taste now and think you cannot beat a bit of lemon juice squeezed over a serving of greens, carrots or fresh beans. You could even try the orange sauce we described above.

Old recipes need not become dead recipes. You can usually **transform your old favourites** into high-LifePoints, low-RiskPoints dishes by performing one or two simple amendments. Here is a recipe rewriting programme we suggest will work with most of your past glories:

1) Does it include pastry? Substitute with New Pastry (page 134).

2) Does it include a sauté stage? Use the New Sauté (page 150).

3) Does it include eggs? If for texture and colour, use mashed tofu and turmeric. If for binding purposes, use a little agar powder, breadcrumbs or a tablespoon of rice flakes. If for raising purposes, use egg substitute plus an agent such as baking powder, as appropriate.

4) Does it include fish? Try using Quorn instead, available from most supermarkets.

5) Does it include fatty meat? Use textured vegetable protein (TVP) or a product such as VegeMince instead. This is now widely available, both from supermarkets and health food shops, and is available in mince and chunk form. It is also available in plain, beef or chicken flavours. As you can see from the listings (see 'Meat substitute' in the Legumes section), TVP is very high in LifePoints and definitely counts as one of our value-added foods.

6)   Does it include milk? Use skimmed milk or soya milk, or substitute another liquid such as fruit juice or vegetable stock.

7)   'Does it include cream? Usually low-fat plain yogurt will do instead.

8)   Does it include cheese? First, reduce the amount asked for by three-quarters, adding rice flakes or lentils to make up for the texture and binding qualities. Second, try eliminating it entirely and use tofu or nutritional yeast flakes instead (available from health food shops).

9)   Does it include sugar? Try using a small amount of blackstrap molasses instead. Whilst adding its own definite flavour, it also adds a few LifePoints, which sugar sadly lacks.

10)   Is it deep-fried? Sorry, find a new favourite! Deep-frying, in our language, is the same as deep trouble.

You might need to spend a little longer cooking during the first few weeks on the LifePoints Diet. We hope you enjoy it! It's not often that one gets a chance to take a fresh look at the way one does things and, in this case, we know the outcome will be delicious and rewarding. To help you plan your menus and your cooking time, however, we include a few tips here, some of which you might already be familiar with:

- Cook a giant pot of soup on Sunday evening and freeze it in lunch-sized servings. Take one out of the freezer every morning and reheat it at work. For more soup recipes, see the *LifePoints Cookbook*.
- Most beans and vegetables can be cooked and then marinated all day or overnight for a really exquisite flavour. We offer some specific recipes in the *LifePoints Cookbook*. The beauty of these marinades is that they may be stored, covered, in the fridge and used as snacks, salads or lunches for the next 3–4 days. All are high in LifePoints and, if you make the marinade oil-free, low in RiskPoints too.
- Practice this quick assessment to help you judge whether the meal you plan is going to provide foods from a variety of food groups:

1)   Fill half the plate with potatoes or rice, buckwheat, millet or other grain.

2) Fill one quarter of the plate with green vegetables.
3) Fill one quarter of the plate with yellow-orange vegetables.
4) Use only no-fat or low-fat sauces, gravies and dressings.
5) Let dessert be fruit.

Of course, all these colours and foods can be mixed, as they naturally are in a salad or pilaf, for instance.

● Prepare a grain or lentil loaf (see the *LifePoints Cookbook*) and slice leftovers into sandwiches and salads during the next 2–3 days.

Finally, add zero-RiskPoints, high-LifePoints foods freely to enhance your enjoyment of each meal and snack. Most people find the quantity of food listed in each menu more than ample but adding LifePoints-only foods will ensure you don't get hungry and that, if you feel a snack coming on, you have plenty of options from which to choose. The listings in Part Five give you plenty of examples.

EXERCISE YOUR LIFESTYLE

We recommend that you exercise, in some form, every day of your life. Exercise, like eating well, is a natural and instinctive part of being human which has sadly been overtaken by the modern lifestyle. But, like eating well, it can be rediscovered. As part of the LifePoints Diet, we included the Kick-Start to help you get on track for a new lifestyle. Now we urge you to continue on that track and to proceed with the Walk One Mile challenge and the Kick-Start Stretches. At the end of six weeks, if you feel you want more success in your life, extend your fitness routine to include another form of exercise. Our view is that walking and stretching are the essentials that should not disappear from your life; games, classes, dance and all the many other forms of exercise should be used as bonuses to further enhance your fitness and your enjoyment of your life. Select them carefully and practise them happily and safely. Good luck.

MORE ABOUT EXERCISE

'Exercise is good for you!' True or false? In fact, only a kind of exercise suited to your age, physical state, interests and budget can really be good for you. And exercise is an exact science; there are certain kinds of physical activity that your body needs, and others that it certainly does not. Exercise is really just a way of challenging your body to function at its best while moving and breathing. Of course, it is often associated with games, sports and very hard work, but it needn't include any of these. All it need be is a time and activity specially set aside for you to enjoy using your body. Regular exercise helps to:

- keep your weight normalized
- keep your joints flexible
- keep your muscles strong and elastic
- keep your cardio-respiratory system (heart/lungs) healthy
- keep your posture well aligned
- maintain good circulation
- improve skin tone
- reduce stress
- lift your spirits and improve self-esteem
- minimize the discomfort and progress of some disorders, such as rheumatoid arthritis and osteoporosis
- boost your level of energy
- improve the quality and/or length of your sleep.

Here is a little more information about exercising which we hope will help you fit it permanently into your lifestyle. These notes are broad, for all forms of exercise, and though they may read, at first, like words of caution they are necessary to ensure you understand how emphatic the effect of exercise can be.

Take Care

If you exercise regularly, the fitness you acquire will enable you to do more exercise more safely than when you first started. If you're doing more than you're currently fit for, however, your body has a number of ways of letting you know. Slow or temporarily stop your exercise if:

- You get so breathless you cannot speak.
- You feel pain of any sort anywhere in your body. There is a difference between a mild muscular discomfort sometimes felt while exercising and real pain. So, a 'stitch' or cramp will

cause you to stop for a moment, but you can start up again more gently after a moment's break. Trust your body's pain reflex – it's there to protect you from damage.

- You still feel 'puffed', have a pounding heart or racing pulse more than ten minutes after stopping. This is a definite sign that you should be doing less. Remember, improvement is gradual.
- Discomfort in the joints lasts more than a couple of hours after you've stopped, or if your joints feel worse, not better, the next day. If you have joint problems, exercise can improve their condition, but you may have an initial few days of discomfort.

Stop at once and let your doctor know if you experience chest pain or pressure, dizziness, fainting or visible facial pallor.

Avoiding Injury

- If you take regular medication, or if your general health is poor, then ask your doctor about suitable forms of exercise.
- Make sure a drink of water is nearby when you exercise. The older you get the more prone you are to dehydration. Avoid perspiration-inducing rubberized clothing for this same reason.
- If your exercise is an outdoor activity, avoid exercising in temperature extremes. With age, especially, you are more prone to excessive heat loss in cold weather and to over-heating in the sun.
- Do not begin active or strenuous exercise until at least one hour after a meal.
- Don't exercise on concrete or asphalt. Surfaces with a bit of natural 'give', like wood or grass, will jar your limbs much less, as well as being less painful and injurious if you fall.
- Wear shoes which cushion your feet. Add a good insole if necessary, or you will transmit undue shock to weight-bearing joints.

Enjoy Your Exercise!

Misery is bad for your health. Select a type of exercise that you enjoy the look and feel of, one that fits in with other aspects of your lifestyle. A little trial and error here will make all the difference, so allow yourself a month or so to experiment with different classes and activities. When you find one or more that you like, schedule them into your life so that you can enjoy them with gusto. How do you decide which exercises will suit you? First, you need to be aware that to really benefit you, exercise should cause:

- Your muscles to both stretch and contract. As well as improving your shape and establishing strength and endurance, developed muscle tissue is necessary to support your joints and internal organs. Many serious health problems arise out of poor muscle tone, such as hernia, back problems, prolapse and digestive problems.
- All your major joints to move. Movement stimulates the circulation of blood and lymph and keeps the joints mobile.
- You to breathe deeply and regularly, perhaps becoming *slightly* breathless though still able to talk. Many kinds of exertion have this effect, but you need to keep yourself exercising to this level for several minutes to benefit your cardiovascular system. Exercising to this level helps to keep blood pressure down, arteries clear, and heart and lungs strong and healthy. If you under-exert yourself you do not gain fitness; and over-exertion to the point of breathlessness does not improve fitness either and can lead to serious problems such as a heart attack.
- Your heart to pump strongly and regularly. You should monitor this by watching your breathing, as above. Do not allow yourself to go red in the face, dizzy, or to feel the thumping of your heart in your ears! In any form of exercise, you must remain in charge. Don't be bullied or feel you have to keep up. If in any doubt, *stop*.
- Your brain to deal with co-ordination or movement patterns. This aspect of exercise creates opportunity for relaxation, stress reduction, creativity and fun. No exercise should be without these.

In addition, an exercise only really suits you if:

- It is enjoyable and affordable.
- You can practice it at least three times each week.

- It includes warm up and cool down movements in each session.
- It is interesting to you, so that you welcome its practice as a regular feature in your daily life.

Which Exercise?

Pick an exercise after first deciding what sort of practice schedule and environment best suits you. For instance, would you prefer:

- A group exercise such as a game or class *or* a solitary exercise?
- A morning-only, daytime-only, evening-only, etc, exercise session?
- An exercise that is silent *or* accompanied by rhythmic music?
- Exercise that involves a little expense, to keep you motivated?
- Excrcise that is free except for the clothes you will wear?
- A strict routine *or* a lot of variety?
- Three or four seasonal exercises *or* one year-round exercise?

Here are basic evaluations of some of the more common forms of exercise. The summary for each exercise follows the format:

- Where or how is it done?
- For how long is it done?
- Why or for whom is it especially beneficial?
- What are its special attractions?
- What are the clothing requirements?
- What are the drawbacks or disadvantages?

AEROBICS

- Indoors with an instructor; many sports centres, church halls
- 15 minutes excluding warm up and cool down, average total of 45–60 minutes
- Challenges the cardiovascular system, best for the youngish and fairly fit
- Very social, usually to music and can be quite dance-like
- Minimum of loose or stretchy clothing with good training shoes
- Quality of exercise dependent on quality of teacher, also some floors are too hard for this exercise and injury can result.

Cycling

- Indoors on a stationary bicycle *or* outdoors on a geared bicycle
- Minimum of 20 minutes without stopping
- Especially good for the elderly or those with hip or back problems
- Little likelihood of injury to muscle, tendon, ligament, etc.
- Wear non-chafe clothing and a helmet for outdoor cycling
- Outdoor cyclists should plan a safe, non-stop route with few hills.

Dancing

- Ballroom, rock 'n'roll, disco, folk, Scottish country or any other
- Minimum of 12 minutes without a complete break
- Very social and pleasant for those who like music and rhythm
- An attractive activity which makes one feel competent and controlled
- Wear flat, comfortable shoes to avoid foot injury
- Dance with a partner who can also dance for 12 minutes or try line-dancing which is partnerless.
- SPECIAL NOTE: dancing is something you can do in your own home to your favourite music whenever you like. It's nice to have a partner, but it's not essential. Dancing includes any movement that feels graceful or rhythmical to you – it doesn't have to comply with anyone else's idea of a dance! *Any* movement you make helps to exercise your joints and muscles, so all of it does you some good.

Games

- Volleyball, squash, tennis, golf or similar
- Minimum of 30 minutes, as these are usually stop-start activities
- Especially good for those who like to compete or follow a set of rules
- Social yet with a chance for individual accomplishment and skill
- Wear shoes and clothing suited to the game, allowing free movement
- Play with a partner who will challenge you, but not too much.

JARMING

- Sitting in a chair and 'jogging' with your arms
- Minimum of 15 minutes without stopping
- Particularly for those who are elderly or in any way infirm
- Achieves cardio-respiratory goals safely and effectively
- May be performed to rhythmic music
- Maintain a size and pace of 'jarm' that will allow adequate breath
- SPECIAL NOTE: most jarmers find it more fun if they jarm to rhythmic music, or 'conduct' their favourite symphonic music.

JOGGING

- In an indoor court *or* outdoors on track or field
- Minimum of 15 minutes without stopping
- For those who are able to exercise strenuously without pain
- May be social or solitary with scope for competition if desired
- Select very supportive shoes and non-chafe clothing
- Weather, dogs and mud are always hazards.

KEEP FIT

- In a class or at home using an audio cassette or video tape
- Minimum of 30 minutes, including warm up and cool down
- For a complete fitness programme of stretch, strength and mobility
- For all ages; classes are usually very social and full of variety
- Wear loose or stretchy clothing
- Make sure your teacher is qualified and gives you personal attention.

ROWING

- On an indoor machine *or* join an outdoor rowing club
- Minimum of 15 minutes without stopping
- An excellent way to exercise the whole body
- For all ages; having particular effect on arms, legs, back and abdomen
- Wear minimum, non-chafe clothing
- Indoors, select a machine with a comfortable, sliding seat.

SKIING OR SKATING

- Cross-country skiing *or* ice skating *or* roller skating
- Minimum of 20 minutes without stopping
- All the benefits of running or jogging
- Mostly lower-body exercise, though arm movement improves breathing
- Wear stretchy, non-chafe clothing and appropriate skis or skates
- Skiing is seasonal, and you need to find rink space for skating.

SWIMMING

- In this country, usually an indoor exercise
- Minimum of 20 minutes without stopping
- Excellent to loosen joints and muscles and improve heart and lungs
- A variety of strokes ensure the majority of joints and muscles are used
- Wear minimum clothing
- Finding a clean, uncrowded pool is sometimes difficult
- SPECIAL NOTE: swimming is an excellent all-body exercise, good for people of advanced years, or with advanced osteoporosis and other disorders that make weight-bearing exercise difficult. In fact, because the water supports your weight, swimming can make you feel that all your physical impediments have temporarily vanished, at the same time as exercising all your muscles. Most swimming pools have cheaper rates for pensioners, and many have special sessions for the over-fifties or sixties. These are great fun, child-free and full of new people to meet.

WALKING

- An anywhere, anytime activity
- Minimum of 20 minutes without stopping
- An excellent exercise for heart, lungs, back and lower body
- For all ages
- Wear high-quality supportive shoes
- It is necessary to maintain a brisk pace for maximum benefit.

WEIGHT TRAINING

- Using a multi-gym or poly-gym arrangement in a sports centre

- Aim for 20–30 minutes of sustained training
- Improves strength, muscle tone and posture in specific body parts
- For all ages; provides an opportunity to become more physically aware
- Wear supportive shoes and loose or stretchy clothing
- A qualified coach is essential in your first month of training.

YOGA

- At home from memory *or* at a class run by a certified teacher
- Most classes last at least one hour, some up to two and a half hours
- Increases your mobility, suppleness, posture and improves breathing
- For all ages; also gives you time and mental space to contemplate
- Wear loose or stretchy clothing and have an extra layer at hand
- It can take time to find the teacher and type of yoga class that suit you
- SPECIAL NOTE: though not at all a yoga practice, we thought we should mention t'ai chi, an ancient oriental form of martial art used as an exercise by millions of people of all ages, sizes and levels of fitness. T'ai chi is a series of slow movements designed to keep your *chi* (energy) flowing properly; it is believed to prolong health into great old age and is certainly an excellent way to stay limber without making excessive demands on your body. Check your local paper or library for the nearest class.

Precautions
Do NOT exercise if:
- You are ill
- You are injured
- You are undernourished
- You are *very* tired, physically, mentally or emotionally
- You have already exercised strenuously that day
- You have a medical condition which requires a doctor's advice – get his or her opinion on the exercise programme you wish to follow.

Double Check

If you have an idea you would like to do a particular form of exercise, attend one session before you enrol for a course or spend out on expensive equipment. Look for a new teacher if you find that:

- You're not given the opportunity to warm up and cool down properly.
- You're pushed straight into complex exercises you don't understand.
- You're not taught the correct details of the movements, leaving you confused and your muscles hurting before the session ends.

If you like the teacher, the place and, so far, the type of exercise, decide finally if it is an appropriate exercise for you by asking yourself the following questions:

- Will it make my heart and lungs work hard but not too hard? Remember – you want to be just *slightly* breathless.
- Will it tone my muscles and make me move all major joints?
- Will I be able to do it regularly? Half an hour, three to five times a week is a good average.
- Does it require a bit of brain work in the form of co-ordination or remembering movement patterns?
- Will I enjoy it?
- Does it suit my age and current level of health and fitness?

How to start

Always take a safe and sensible route into your exercise programme:

- Discuss with your doctor your intention to begin an exercise programme or take up a new activity.
- Select a form of exercise that really suits you.
- Begin slowly and extend your practice gradually.
- Set yourself a daily target that you know is comfortably within your scope. Practise that amount every day for a week or two, then try extending your practice over several weeks until you arrive at a level of exercise you feel happy doing. When

walking, for instance, you might try adding 10 per cent to the distance every other week until you reach a pace and distance you are very happy with.

Keeping It Up

- If you stop enjoying your exercise, find a new one to replace it.
- Practise your exercise at a regular time, whenever possible, so that it becomes an important part of your day. Ideally, you should really regret missing a session.
- Most forms of exercise are stimulating, so try not to do yours just before bedtime.
- A supportive partner or friend, joining in or just applauding, is usually an encouragement to continue your exercise.
- Have one or two exercise options up your sleeve if, for any reason, you can't practise your favourite form. This way you won't lose the place in your schedule reserved for exercise.
- Keep an exercise diary: chances are that if you record several days' neglect these will coincide with several days of lethargy, depression, aches and pains, and so on.
- Practise two or three different forms of exercise in rotation to keep variety in your life.
- Ask that your birthday and Christmas gifts, etc, be things such as clothing, musical cassettes or equipment that you can use in your exercise sessions.

Exercise for Life!

There is an old saying 'If you don't have time for exercise, you'll certainly have time for illness'. Exercise helps to keep you well. Get to know and like two or three different types of exercise and simply rotate your practice of them to keep yourself interested and active. We hope that these notes will help you establish a programme of exercise that suits you precisely, one that you can enjoy – and that will benefit you – for years to come.

Evaluate Your LifeStyle

Hopefully you have kept a diet diary for the duration of the Kick-Start. This isn't easy or natural for everyone but it is useful for you to have a record of a few starting points from which you might gain motivation or a feeling of achievement. Here is how we suggest you use these notes:

- Weigh yourself every week for the first three months of the LifePoints diet and compare this weight with that measured on Day One and Day Seven. After three to six months, weigh yourself about once each month but no less than every year – why not on your birthday!

- Use the notes you have made on frequency and duration of exercise to chart, at least mentally, your success and achievement at your chosen form of exercise. And use your notes on various forms of exercise you may have tried to fine-tune your practice so that you arrive at a routine you really enjoy.

- If you have noted chronic or long-standing health problems or disorders, you may notice that these have gradually diminished in importance or incidence during the first six weeks of using the LifePoints system. In fact, it is useful for some people to remind themselves that these problems even existed as they, quite rightly, push them rather quickly from their thoughts. In any case, noting an increasing sense of well-being will provide incentive and motivation for continuing a good diet and an exercise routine.

- Having made notes of your starting point in terms of fitness and exercise, you should be rightly proud of the achievements you have made. It is useful to make notes and then compare these notes at Day One, Day Seven and then monthly for a year or two. Some people cannot Walk One Mile on Day One but they can during Week Three and they can Walk One Mile in 20 minutes during the third month. These are great achievements and they are made remarkable by the fact that you note your starting point and proceed determinedly from there.

- Finally, the notes you made on specific foods, cookery, menu planning or any other aspect of the Kick-Start will benefit you now or later when you decide to try a new food or recipe. A process of continuous evaluation of your diet and exercise programme will always benefit you, whether or not it is in note form. As various aspects of your life change, you will need to amend your diet and lifestyle to preserve optimum health. LifePoints is about evaluating your diet, first and foremost, and we hope it will put years on your life – and lots of life into your years!

PART FIVE: FOOD TO COUNT ON

The LifePoints Diet is all about freedom – the freedom to eat according to your own personal tastes, not according to the likes or dislikes of diet book authors! That's why – at the heart of the LifePoints system – lies the counter, a unique listing of food divided into six major groups (remember, the first four are compulsory, the last two optional). The LifePoints food control system is very powerful, and can be used in a number of ways. For example, you can use it to analyse your existing diet and see where the holes are. You can use it to plan a really healthy diet, following the guidelines explained in Part Two of this book. Or – the easiest way of all – you can simply use the system to check out the difference between two foods to find the healthiest! One thing is certain – as you glance through the foods that follow, you'll never see them in quite the same way again. We hope you share the thrill we first felt when you realize just how effective and uncomplicated the LifePoints system is to use. Sheer power over your diet . . . at your fingertips!

THE TOP TEN LIFEPOINTS POWER FOODS
People often ask us to nominate our 'top ten' foods from each of the four essential groups. Here they are, together with their associated RiskPoints and LifePoints . . .

GROUP ONE: FRUIT AND FRUIT JUICES

Food	RiskPoints ✘	LifePoints ✔
Papaya: fresh	1	12
Melon: cantaloupe	1	10
Orange juice: fresh	1	9
Guavas: fresh	2	9
Pineapple juice	0	8
Apricots: dehydrated	0	8
Prunes: dehydrated	1	7
Mangos: fresh	1	7
Figs: dried	2	7
Bananas: fresh	1	6

GROUP TWO: CEREALS, GRAINS AND PASTA

Food	RiskPoints ✘	LifePoints ✔
Raisin bran	1	32
Grape Nuts	0	23
All Bran	1	22
Semolina	2	18
Wheat germ: toasted	7	18
Soya flour: low-fat	7	17
Corn flakes	0	16
Porridge: made with skimmed milk	5	13
Millet: cooked	6	12
Pizza: with tomatoes and olives, no cheese	8	10

GROUP THREE: VEGETABLES AND VEGETABLE PRODUCTS

Food	RiskPoints ✗	LifePoints ✔
Spinach: steamed	1	25
Baked potato topped with baked beans	1	20
Asparagus: canned	4	18
Turnip greens: boiled	0	16
Broccoli: fresh	1	14
Beansprouts: stir-fried	0	11
Yeast extract: fortified with vitamin B12	0	11
Squash: baked	3	10
Vegetables: mixed, canned	1	10
Green beans: canned	0	10

GROUP FOUR: LEGUMES, NUTS AND SEEDS

Food	RiskPoints ✗	LifePoints ✔
Textured vegetable protein (TVP)	2	21
Baked beans: on toast, no butter	4	17
Lentils: boiled	0	16
Adzuki beans: boiled	0	13
Kidney beans: boiled	1	12
Chick peas: boiled	5	12
Bean pâté: made with lentils	0	11
Peas: split, boiled	0	9
Broadbeans: boiled	0	9
Ginkgo nuts: dried	1	6

GROUP ONE: FRUIT AND FRUIT JUICES

	RiskPoints ✗	LifePoints ✔
Apples: dried, sulphured, uncooked (5 rings/32g) 78 cals	0	1
Apples: fresh with skin (1 fruit/ 138g) 81 cals	1	1
Apples: fresh without skin (1 fruit/128g) 73 cals	0	1
Apples: juice, canned or bottled, without added vitamin C (1 cup/ 8 fl oz/248g) 117 cals	0	1
Apple sauce: canned, unsweetened without added vitamin C (½ cup/ 122g) 52 cals	0	1
Apricot nectar: canned, without added vitamin C (1 cup/8fl oz/ 251g) 141 cals	0	3
Apricots: dehydrated (low-moisture) sulphured, un-cooked (½ cup/60g) 192 cals	0	8
Apricots: dried, sulphured, uncooked (10 halves/35g) 83 cals	0	3
Apricots: fresh (3 fruits/106g) 51 cals	1	3
Avocado: see the Vegetables and Vegetable Products section		
Bananas: fresh (1 fruit/114g) 105 cals	1	6
Blackberries: fresh (1 cup/144g) 75 cals	1	6
Blackberries: frozen unsweetened (1 cup/151g) 97 cals	1	7
Blackcurrants: fresh (½ cup/56g) 35 cals	0	2

	RiskPoints ✗	LifePoints ✔
Blueberries: fresh (1 cup/145g) 81 cals	1	3
Cherries: sour red, fresh (1 cup with stones/103g) 52 cals	0	2
Cherries: sweet, fresh (1 cup/ 145g) 104 cals	3	3
Cranberry: fresh (1 cup whole/ 95g) 47 cals	0	1
Cranberry: juice cocktail (1 cup/ 8 fl oz/253g) 144 cals	0	2
Cranberry: sauce, canned, sweetened (½ cup/138g) 208 cals	0	1
Cranberry-apple juice drink (1 cup/8 fl oz/245g) 164 cals	0	2
Currants: zante, dried (½ cup/ 72g) 204 cals	0	6
Dates: fresh and dry (10 fruits/ 83g) 228 cals	0	5
Figs: dried, uncooked (5 fruits/ 93g) 237 cals	2	7
Figs: fresh (1 medium fruit/50g) 37 cals	0	1
Gooseberries: fresh (½ cup/75g) 33 cals	1	2
Granadilla: *see* 'Passion-fruit'		
Grape juice: canned or bottled, unsweetened (1 cup/8 fl oz/ 253g) 154 cals	0	3
Grapefruit: fresh (½ fruit/120g) 38 cals	0	2
Grapefruit juice: canned, unsweetened (1 cup/8 fl oz/ 247g) 94 cals	0	4

	RiskPoints ✗	LifePoints ✔
Grapes: fresh (10 fruits/50g) 36 cals	0	1
Guava sauce: cooked (½ cup/119g) 43 cals	0	3
Guavas: fresh (1 cup/165g) 84 cals	2	9
Kiwi fruit (Chinese gooseberries): fresh (1 medium fruit/76g) 46 cals	0	2
Kumquats: fresh (4 fruits/80g) 50 cals	0	3
Lemon juice: canned or bottled (1 cup/8 fl oz/244g) 51 cals	1	4
Lemon juice: fresh (1 cup/8 fl oz/244g) 61 cals	0	5
Lemons: fresh, without peel (1 medium fruit/58g) 17 cals	0	1
Lime juice: canned or bottled, unsweetened (1 cup/8 fl oz/246g) 52 cals	1	3
Lime juice: fresh (1 cup/8 fl oz/246g) 66 cals	0	3
Limes: fresh (1 fruit 2 in diam/67g) 20 cals	0	1
Lychees: fresh (1 cup/190g) 125 cals	2	4
Mangos: fresh (1 fruit/207g) 135 cals	1	7
Melons: cantaloupe, fresh (½ fruit/267g) 93 cals	1	10
Melons: honeydew, fresh (1 cup cubed pieces/170g) 60 cals	0	3
Nectarines: fresh (1 fruit/136g) 67 cals	1	2

	RiskPoints ✗	LifePoints ✔
Orange and apricot juice drink: (1 cup/8 fl oz/250g) 128 cals	0	3
Orange juice: canned, unsweetened (1 cup/8 fl oz/249g) 105 cals	0	7
Orange juice: fresh (1 cup/8 fl oz/248g) 112 cals	1	9
Orange juice: fresh (juice from 1 fruit/86g) 39 cals	0	3
Orange juice: made from concentrate (1 cup/8 fl oz/249g) 110 cals	1	7
Oranges: fresh (1 fruit/131g) 62 cals	0	6
Papayas: fresh (1 fruit/304g) 119 cals	1	12
Passion-fruit: fresh (1 fruit/18g) 17 cals	0	0
Passion-fruit juice: fresh (1 cup/8 fl oz/247g) 126 cals	0	5
Peach nectar: canned without added vitamin C (1 cup/8 fl oz/249g) 134 cals	0	2
Peaches: dried, sulphured, uncooked (5 halves/65g) 155 cals	1	5
Peaches: fresh (1 fruit/4 per lb/87g) 37 cals	0	1
Pear nectar: canned without added vitamin C (1 cup/8 fl oz/250g) 150 cals	0	1
Pears: dried, sulphured, uncooked (5 halves/87g) 228 cals	1	4
Pears: fresh (1 fruit/166g) 98 cals	1	2

	RiskPoints ✗	LifePoints ✔
Pineapple: fresh (1 slice 3½ in diam/84g) 41 cals	0	2
Pineapple juice: canned, unsweetened without added vitamin C (1 cup/8 fl oz/250g) 140 cals	0	7
Plantain: cooked (½ cup slices/ 77g) 89 cals	0	3
Plums: fresh (1 fruit 2⅛ in diam/ 66g) 36 cals	1	1
Pomegranate: fresh (1 fruit 3⅜ in diam/154g) 105 cals	1	2
Pomelo: fresh (1 fruit/609g) 231 cals	0	11
Prickly pears: fresh (1 fruit/103g) 42 cals	1	2
Prune juice: canned (1 cup/8fl oz/256g) 182 cals	0	8
Prunes: dehydrated (low-moisture) stewed (½ cup/140g) 158 cals	0	4
Prunes: dehydrated (low-moisture) uncooked (½ cup/66g) 224 cals	1	7
Prunes: dried, uncooked (5 fruits without stones/42g) 100 cals	0	3
Quinces: fresh (1 fruit/92g) 52 cals	0	1
Raisins: seedless (½ cup packed/ 82g) 246 cals	0	5
Raspberries: fresh (1 cup/123g) 60 cals	1	6
Raspberries: frozen (½ cup/125g) 129 cals	0	4
Redcurrants: fresh (½ cup/56g) 31 cals	0	1

	RiskPoints ✗	LifePoints ✓
Soursop: fresh (½ fruit/312g) 206 cals	2	9
Starfruit: fresh (1 fruit without seeds/127g) 42 cals	1	2
Strawberries: fresh (1 cup/149g) 45 cals	1	5
Sultanas: (½ cup packed/82g) 248 cals	0	5
Tamarinds: fresh (1 fruit/2g) 5 cals	0	0
Tangerines: fresh (1 fruit/84g) 37 cals	0	3
Watermelon: fresh (1/16 fruit/ 482g) 154 cals	5	10
Whitecurrants: fresh (½ cup/56g) 31 cals	0	1

GROUP TWO: CEREALS, GRAINS AND PASTA

Breakfast Cereals

The average weight of most servings of breakfast cereals is about 1oz (28g): first choose your cereal, then add either whole, semi-skimmed, skimmed or soya milk as below.	RiskPoints ✗	LifePoints ✔
40% bran flakes: (1 oz/28g) 93 cals	1	32
100% toasted wheat bran sticks (1oz/28g) 71 cals	1	22
Corn flakes: honey and nut (1oz/28g) 113 cals	3	16
Corn flakes: regular (1oz/28g) 110 cals	0	16
Corn flakes: sugar frosted (1oz/28g) 108 cals	0	16
Crispy wheat and raisins: (1oz/28g) 99 cals	1	20
Frosted rice crispies: (1oz/28g) 109 cals	0	16
Grape Nuts: (1oz/28g) 101 cals	0	23
Muesli: homemade, oats with wheat germ and nuts (1 oz/28g) 138 cals	19	5
Oat flakes: fortified (1oz/28g) 105 cals	1	27
Raisin bran: (1.3oz/36g) 115 cals	1	32
Shreds of wheat: large biscuit (2 biscuits/38g) 133 cals	1	6
Shreds of wheat: small biscuits (1oz/28g) 102 cals	1	5
Special low-calorie rice and wheat flakes: (1oz/28g) 111 cals	0	21
Sugary corn smacks: (1oz/28g) 106 cals	1	16

	RiskPoints ✗	LifePoints ✔
Pressed wheat flakes: (2 biscuits/ 28g) 95 cals	2	9
Wheat germ: toasted, plain (1oz/ 28g) 108 cals	7	18

	RiskPoints ✗	LifePoints ✔
Milk: cow's, whole (the serving size for a bowl of cereal is about ¾ cup/183g) 117 cals	31	9
Milk: cow's, semi-skimmed (¾ cup/183g) 101 cals	16	10
Milk: cow's, skimmed (¾ cup/ 183g) 64 cals	1	9
Milk: soya (¾ cup/183g) 60 cals	8	5

Cooked Breakfast Foods

For egg dishes, such as omelettes, hard-boiled eggs, etc. see Eggs in the Meat, Fish and Dairy group	RiskPoints ✗	LifePoints ✔
Cream of rice: cooked with water (¾ cup/183g) 95 cals	0	1
Cream of wheat: cooked with water (¾ cup/188g) 100 cals	0	7
French toast: with butter (2 slices/135g) 356 cals	58	15
Instant oats: fortified, plain, prepared with water (1 serving/ 177g) 104 cals	·4	25
Instant oats: fortified, with apples and cinnamon, prepared with water (1 serving/149g) 136 cals	4	23
Muffin: blueberry, prepared with whole milk (1 muffin/57g) 165 cals	16	5
Muffin: plain, prepared with whole milk (1 muffin/57g) 172 cals	17	6

	RiskPoints ✗	LifePoints ✔
Pancakes: plain (1 pancake/38g) 86 cals	9	3
Pancakes: made with blueberries (1 pancake/38g) 84 cals	8	3
Pancakes: with butter and syrup (3 pancakes/232g) 520 cals	43	15
Porridge: made with skimmed milk (¾ cup/210g) 168 cals	5	13
Porridge: made with semi-skimmed milk (¾ cup/210g) 205 cals	19	15
Porridge: made with soya milk (¾ cup/207g) 163 cals	12	10
Porridge: made with water (¾ cup/175g) 109 cals	4	4
Porridge: made with whole milk (¾ cup/210g) 221 cals	33	13
Waffles: plain (1 waffle/75g) 218 cals	26	9

Breads

There's an infinite number of breads and bread products in the world, most of which are extremely delicious and very healthy, too. Here we've gathered comprehensive information for many of the most common kinds.	RiskPoints ✗	LifePoints ✔
Bagels: cinnamon-raisin (3½ in bagel/71g) 195 cals	3	8
Bagels: egg (3½ in bagel/71g) 197 cals	3	9
Bagels: plain or with onion, poppy or sesame seed (3½ in bagel/71g) 195 cals	2	10

	RiskPoints ✗	LifePoints ✔
Banana bread: made with margarine (1 slice/60g) 196 cals	15	3
Banana bread: made with vegetable shortening (1 slice/60g) 203 cals	17	3
Breadcrumbs: dry, grated, plain (1oz/28g) 112 cals	3	6
Bread sticks: plain (1 stick/10g) 41 cals	2	1
Chapati: (1 medium made without fat/35g) 71 cals	0	2
Cornbread: made with low-fat milk (1 piece/65g) 173 cals	11	7
Croissant: apple (1 croissant/57g) 145 cals	18	4
Croissant: with butter (1 croissant/57g) 231 cals	50	6
Croissant: cheese (1 croissant/57g) 236 cals	41	8
Croissant: chocolate (1 croissant/72g) 310 cals	86	8
Croissant: with egg, cheese and ham (1 croissant/152g) 474 cals	131	20
Croûtons (¼ cup/7g) 31 cals	1	1
Crumpet: plain, toasted (1 crumpet/52g) 133 cals	2	6
Crumpet: with butter (1 crumpet/57g) 169 cals	20	6
Dinner roll: wholewheat (1 roll/28g) 75 cals	3	3
Dumplings: (2 average/60g) 127 cals	29	2
Egg bread: (brioche) (1 slice/40g) 115 cals	6	6

	RiskPoints ✗	LifePoints ✔
French bread: (1 medium slice/25g) 69 cals	1	3
French roll: (1 roll/38g) 105 cals	4	5
Granary: toasted (1 slice/25g) 73 cals	2	3
Hamburger or hotdog buns: (1 bun/43g) 123 cals	5	5
Irish soda bread: (1 slice/60g) 174 cals	7	5
Italian bread: (1 slice/30g) 81 cals	2	4
Pitta: white (1 pitta/60g) 165 cals	1	8
Pitta: wholewheat (1 pitta/64g) 170 cals	4	8
Pizza: with cheese (1 slice–⅛th of a pizza/63g) 140 cals	11	11
Pizza: with cheese, meat and vegetables (1 slice–⅛th of a pizza/79g) 184 cals	13	11
Pizza: with pepperoni (1 slice–⅛th of a pizza/71g) 181 cals	17	10
Pizza: with tomatoes and olives, no cheese (1 slice–⅛th of á pizza/63g) 142 cals	8	10
Pumpernickel: (1 slice/32g) 80 cals	2	4
Raisin bread: (1 slice/26g) 71 cals	2	3
Rye bread: (1 slice/32g) 83 cals	2	4
Scones: plain or buttermilk (1 scone/35g) 127 cals	14	3
Toast: with butter, made with wholewheat bread (1 slice/30g) 105 cals	27	3
Toast: with margarine, made with wholewheat bread (1 slice/30g) 105 cals	13	3

	RiskPoints ✗	LifePoints ✔
Toast: with olive oil, made with wholewheat bread and 1 teaspoon olive oil (1 serving/30g) 113 cals	15	3
Vienna bread: *see* 'French bread'		
White bread: soft (1 slice/25g) 67 cals	2	3
White bread: roll (1 roll/28g) 77 cals	4	3
White bread: toasted (1 slice/23g) 67 cals	2	3
Whole wheat bread: soft (1 slice/25g) 62 cals	2	3
Whole wheat bread: toasted (1 slice/25g) 69 cals	3	3
Yorkshire pudding: (1 individual pudding/30g) 65 cals	10	1
Sandwiches and burgers: For a wide selection of popular sandwiches and burgers, please consult *LifePoints*		

Crackers

For sweet biscuits, see 'Biscuits and Cookies' in the Drinks, Desserts, Snacks and Sauces group.	RiskPoints ✗	LifePoints ✔
Crackers: standard snack-type (4 crackers/14g) 71 cals	10	1
Cream crackers: (1 cracker/3g) 13 cals	0	0
Crispbread: rye (1 wafer/10g) 37 cals	0	1
Matzo: (1 matzo/28g) 112 cals	0	3
Melba toast: (1 toast/5g) 20 cals	0	0
Oatcakes: (1 biscuit/10g) 44 cals	4	1

	RiskPoints ✗	LifePoints ✔
Ricecakes: made with brown rice (1 cake/9g) 35 cals	0	1
Rusk: (1 rusk/10g) 41 cals	1	1
Taco shells: baked (1 medium/ 13g) 61 cals	7	1
Tortillas: ready-to-bake or fry (1 medium 25g) 56 cals	1	2

Grains and Flours

	RiskPoints ✗	LifePoints ✔
Arrowroot flour: (⅓ cup/43g) 154 cals	0	0
Barley: pearled, cooked (1 cup/ 157g) 193 cals	1	8
Bulgur: cooked (1 cup/182g) 151 cals	1	8
Cornmeal: (polenta) wholegrain yellow (½ cup/61g) 221 cals	5	8
Cornstarch: (1 tablespoon/8g) 30 cals	0	0
Couscous: cooked (1 cup/179g) 200 cals	0	6
Couscous: prepared with chick peas and mixed vegetables (1 cup/179g) 208 cals	16	8
Millet: cooked (1 cup/240g) 286 cals	6	12
Oats (½ cup/78g) 303 cals	13	14
Popcorn: see 'Snacks and sweets' in the Drinks, Desserts, Snacks and Sauces group		
Quinoa: (1 cup/170g) 636 cals	24	32
Rice: brown, long-grain, cooked (1 cup/195g) 216 cals	4	7

	RiskPoints ✗	LifePoints ✓
Rice: brown, medium-grain, cooked (1 cup/195g) 218 cals	4	6
Rice: white, glutinous, cooked (1 cup/241 g) 234 cals	1	3
Rice: white, long grain, cooked (1 cup/158g) 205 cals	1	6
Rye flour: medium (½ cup/51g) 181 cals	2	6
Semolina: (½ cup/84g) 302 cals	2	18
Soya flour: low-fat (½ cup stirred/44g) 143 cals	7	17
Wheat bran: crude (2 tablespoons/7g) 15 cals	0	3
Wheat germ: crude (¼ cup/29g) 104 cals	7	16
Wheat germ oil: *see* 'Margarines, Oils and Spreads' in the Drinks, Desserts, Snacks and Sauces group		
White all-purpose wheat flour: (½ cup/62g) 226 cals	1	11
White self-rising wheat flour: enriched (½ cup/62g) 219 cals	1	12
Wholewheat flour: wholegrain (½ cup/60g) 203 cals	2	11
Wild rice: cooked (½ cup/82g) 83 cals	0	4

Pasta

	RiskPoints ✗	LifePoints ✓
Cannelloni: meat-filled (3 shells/300g) 334 cals	42	23
Lasagne: made with mince (1 serving/1 cup/300g) 458 cals	75	34

	RiskPoints ✗	LifePoints ✔
Lasagne: made with textured vegetable protein mince (1 serving 1/cup/300g) 351 cals	25	43
Macaroni: baked with cheese (1 serving/1 cup 200g) 348 cals	74	12
Macaroni: regular, cooked (1 cup/140g) 197 cals	2	7
Macaroni: wholewheat, cooked (1 cup/140g) 174 cals	1	6
Noodles: Chinese chow mein, cooked (1 cup/45g) 237 cals	34	7
Noodles: egg, cooked (1 cup/160g) 213 cals	5	9
Noodles: egg with spinach, cooked (1 cup/160g) 211 cals	6	12
Noodles: Japanese, soba, cooked (1 cup/114g) 113 cals	0	3
Noodles: Japanese, somen, cooked (1 cup/176g) 231 cals	0	2
Pasta e fagioli soup: pasta with beans (1 cup/8 fl oz/253g) 195 cals	12	10
Pasta: made with egg, cooked (1 cup/140g) 182 cals	6	8
Pasta: plain, cooked (1 cup/140g) 183 cals	3	7
Pasta: spinach, cooked (1 cup/140g) 182 cals	3	9
Ravioli: with spinach and cheese filling (1 serving/1 cup/240g) 308 cals	41	21
Risotto: à la Milanaise, with meat (1 serving/1½ cups/225g) 240 cals	35	16

	RiskPoints ✗	LifePoints ✔
Risotto: à la Piemontaise, vegetarian with Parmesan cheese (1 serving/1 cup/150g) 209 cals	36	6
Spaghetti: bolognaise (1 serving/2 cups/410g) 538 cals	57	31
Spaghetti: in four cheeses sauce; Gruyère, fontina, Parmesan and mozzarella (1 serving/2 cups/449g) 1106 cals	384	41
Spaghetti: plain, cooked (1 cup/140g) 197 cals	2	7
Spaghetti: wholewheat, cooked (1 cup/140g) 174 cals	1	6
Spaghetti: with Italian sauce; tomatoes, mushrooms, ham, olive oil (1 serving/2 cups/382g) 466 cals	49	18
Spaghetti: with pesto sauce (1 serving/1 cup/255g) 429 cals	43	16
Spaghetti: with simple tomato sauce, made from tomatoes, onion, garlic, olive oil and green pepper (1 serving/2 cups/322g) 303 cals	27	12

GROUP THREE: VEGETABLES AND VEGETABLE PRODUCTS

	RiskPoints ✗	LifePoints ✔
Alfalfa seeds: sprouted (1 cup/33g) 10 cals	0	2
Artichokes (globe or French): boiled (½ cup hearts/84g) 42 cals	0	5
Asparagus: boiled (½ cup/90g) 22 cals	0	10
Asparagus: canned, drained solids (1 can/248g) 47 cals	4	18
Asparagus: soup, cream of (1 cup/8 fl oz/244g) 85 cals	10	4
Aubergine: boiled (½ cup 1 in cubes/48g) 13 cals	0	1
Aubergine: fried in olive oil (½ cup cubes/63g) 137 cals	35	1
Avocado: fresh (½ fruit/100g) 161 cals	38	9
Avocado: guacamole, dip made with avocados and yogurt (½ cup/138g) 184 cals	40	11
Avocado: vinaigrette (½ fruit with 1 tbsp dressing) 231 cals	57	9
Bamboo shoots: boiled (1 cup ½ in slices/120g) 14 cals	0	2
Bamboo shoots: stir-fried in light oil (1 cup slices/125g) 59 cals	13	2
Beansprouts: mung, fresh (1 cup/104g) 31 cals	0	7
Beansprouts: mung, stir-fried (1 cup/124g) 62 cals	0	11
Beet greens: boiled (1 cup/1 in pieces) 39 cals	0	12
Beetroot: boiled (2 beets/100g) 44 cals	0	6

	RiskPoints ✗	LifePoints ✓
Beetroot: fresh (1 beet/81 g) 35 cals	0	6
Beetroot: pickled (¼ cup slices/ 57g) 37 cals	0	1
Broadbeans: boiled (½ cup/100g) 56 cals	1	7
Broccoli: boiled (1 spear/150g) 42 cals	1	11
Broccoli: fresh (1 spear/151g) 42 cals	1	14
Brussels sprouts: boiled (½ cup/ 78g) 30 cals	0	6
Cabbage: Chinese (bok-choi) boiled (1 cup shredded/170g) 20 cals	0	11
Cabbage: Chinese (bok-choi) fresh (1 cup shredded/70g) 9 cals	0	5
Cabbage: red, boiled (1 cup shredded/150g) 32 cals	0	5
Cabbage: red, fresh (1 cup shredded/70g) 19 cals	0	3
Cabbage: savoy, boiled (1 cup shredded/145g) 35 cals	0	7
Cabbage: savoy, fresh (1 cup shredded/70g) 19 cals	0	5
Cabbage: white, boiled (1 cup shredded/150g) 33 cals	1	5
Cabbage: white, fresh (1 cup shredded/70g) 18 cals	0	3
Carrot juice: canned (6 fl oz/ 184g) 74 cals	0	13
Carrots: baby, fresh (10 medium/ 100g) 38 cals	1	4
Carrots: boiled (½ cup slices/ 78g) 35 cals	0	7

	RiskPoints ✗	LifePoints ✔
Carrots: fresh (1 carrot/72g) 31 cals	0	7
Cauliflower: baked with cheese (1 serving/200g) 226 cals	63	14
Cauliflower: boiled (1 cup 1 in pieces/124g) 29 cals	1	7
Cauliflower: fresh (1 cup 1 in pieces 100g) 25 cals	0	6
Celeriac: boiled (1 cup diced/ 150g) 38 cals	0	3
Celeriac: fresh (1 cup/156g) 61 cals	1	6
Celery: boiled (1 cup diced/150g) 27 cals	0	5
Celery: fresh (2 stalks/80g) 13 cals	0	3
Celery: soup, cream of (1 cup/8 fl oz/244g) 90 cals	13	3
Chard: Swiss, boiled (1 cup chopped/175g) 35 cals	0	9
Chard: Swiss, fresh (2 leaves/96g) 18 cals	0	5
Chicory greens: fresh (1 cup chopped/180g) 41 cals	1	17
Chicory roots: fresh (½ cup 1 in pieces/45g) 33 cals	0	1
Chicory: witloof, fresh (½ cup 45g) 8 cals	0	1
Chips: See 'Potato chips'		
Chives: fresh (1 tbsp chopped/ 3g) 1 cal	0	0
Coleslaw: (½ cup/60g) 41 cals	3	2
Collards: boiled (1 cup chopped/ 128g) 35 cals	0	3

	RiskPoints ✗	LifePoints ✔
Collards: fresh (1 cup chopped/ 36g) 11 cals	0	1
Corn oil: *See* 'Margarines, Oils and Spreads' in the Drinks, Desserts, Snacks and Sauces group		
Corn: sweet, boiled (½ cup kernels/82g) 89 cals	2	5
Corn: sweet, canned, cream style (½ cup/128g) 92 cals	1	6
Corn: sweet, canned in brine, drained solids (½ cup/82g) 66 cals	2	4
Corn: sweet, canned with red and green peppers (½ cup/114g) 86 cals	1	5
Corn: sweet, on the cob with butter (1 ear/146g) 155 cals	16	9
Cornsalad: fresh (1 cup/56g) 12 cals	0	4
Courgette: boiled (½ cup slices/ 90g) 14 cals	0	2
Courgette: fresh (½ cup slices/ 65g) 9 cals	0	2
Cress: garden, fresh (½ cup/25g) 8 cals	0	3
Cucumber: fresh (½ cup slices/ 52g) 7 cals	0	1
Dandelion greens: fresh (½ cup chopped/28g) 13 cals	0	3
Dill pickle: (1 medium/65g) 12 cals	0	0
Endive: fresh (½ cup chopped/ 25g) 4 cals	0	2
Fennel bulb: fresh (1 cup sliced/ 87g) 27 cals	0	3

	RiskPoints ✗	LifePoints ✔
French beans: *See* 'Green beans'		
French fries: *See* 'Potato chips'		
Garlic: fresh (3 cloves/9g) 13 cals	0	1
Gazpacho soup: canned, ready-to-serve (1 cup/8 fl oz/244g) 56 cals	5	5
Ginger root: fresh (5 slices 1 in diameter/11g) 8 cals	0	0
Green beans: boiled (1 cup/125g) 44 cals	0	7
Green beans: canned, drained solids (1 can/262g) 52 cals	0	10
Jerusalem artichokes: (½ cup slices/75g) 57 cals	0	4
Kale: boiled (1 cup chopped/130g) 42 cals	1	8
Kale: fresh (1 cup chopped/67g) 34 cals	1	7
Kohlrabi: (thickened bulb-like stems) fresh (½ cup slices/70g) 19 cals	0	3
Kohlrabi: boiled (½ cup slices/82g) 24 cals	0	3
Lamb's lettuce: *see* 'Cornsalad'		
Lambsquarters (aka goosefoot): boiled (½ cup chopped/90g) 29 cals	1	9
Lambsquarters: fresh (½ cup/50g) 22 cals	1	8
Leek: (bulb and lower leaf-portion) boiled (1 leek/124g) 38 cals	0	4
Leek: (bulb and lower leaf-portion) fresh (½ cup chopped/52g) 32 cals	0	3

	RiskPoints ✗	LifePoints ✔
Leek: soup, cream of leek and potato (1 cup/8 fl oz/250g) 154 cals	20	7
Lettuce: butterhead, includes round types (4 leaves/30g) 4 cals	0	1
Lettuce: cos or romaine (4 inner leaves/40g) 6 cals	0	4
Lettuce: iceberg (4 leaves/80g) 10 cals	0	3
Lotus root: boiled (5 slices/45g) 30 cals	0	2
Mangetout: boiled (½ cup/80g) 34 cals	0	5
Mangetout: fresh (½ cup/72g) 30 cals	0	5
Marrow: see 'Squash'		
Minestrone soup: canned, condensed (½ cup/4 fl oz/123g) 84 cals	6	5
Mixed vegetables: see 'Vegetables, mixed'		
Mushrooms: boiled (½ cup pieces/78g) 21 cals	0	6
Mushrooms: canned, drained solids (½ cup pieces/78g) 19 cals	0	3
Mushrooms: fresh (½ cup pieces/35g) 9 cals	0	3
Mushrooms: soup, cream of (1 cup/8 fl oz/248g) 203 cals	59	8
Mushrooms: soup, regular (1 cup/8 fl oz/253g) 96 cals	12	5
Mustard greens: boiled (½ cup chopped/70g) 11 cals	0	5
Mustard greens: fresh (½ cup chopped/28g) 7 cals	0	4

	RiskPoints ✗	LifePoints ✔
Okra: boiled (½ cup slices/80g) 26 cals	0	5
Olive oil: *see* 'Margarines, Oils and Spreads' in the Drinks, Desserts, Snacks and Sauces group		
Olives: ripe, canned (5 small/ 16g) 18 cals	4	0
Onion rings: breaded, frozen and heated in oven (2 rings/20g) 81 cals	13	1
Onions: boiled (½ cup chopped/ 105g) 46 cals	0	3
Onions: fresh (½ cup chopped/ 80g) 30 cals	0	2
Onions: sautéed in olive oil (½ cup/115g) 135 cals	25	3
Onions: soup, cream of (1 cup/8 fl oz/244g) 107 cals	13	2
Onions: soup, regular (1 cup/8 fl oz/241g) 58 cals	4	3
Onions: spring (includes tops and bulb) fresh (½ cup chopped/50g) 16 cals	0	3
Parsley: fresh (½ cup chopped/ 30g) 11 cals	0	5
Parsnips: boiled (½ cup slices/ 78g) 63 cals	0	5
Parsnips: fresh (½ cup slices/ 67g) 50 cals	0	4
Pea soup: condensed, made with equal amount of water (1 cup/8 fl oz/250g) 165 cals	14	6
Peas and carrots: frozen package, boiled (½ cup/80g) 38 cals	0	6
Peas: canned (½ cup/85g) 59 cals	0	6

	RiskPoints ✗	LifePoints ✔
Peas: fresh (½ cup/72g) 58 cals	0	8
Peas: fresh, boiled (½ cup/80g) 67 cals	0	9
Peas: frozen, then boiled (½ cup/ 80g) 62 cals	0	8
Peppers: hot chilli, green, fresh (1 pepper/45g) 18 cals	0	4
Peppers: hot chilli, red, fresh (1 pepper/45g) 18 cals	0	5
Peppers: stuffed with rice and lamb filling plus tomato sauce (1 pepper/330g) 289 cals	32	21
Peppers: stuffed with vegetable filling and tomato sauce (1 pepper/354g) 218 cals	35	19
Peppers: sweet, green, boiled (1 pepper/73g) 20 cals	0	3
Peppers: sweet, green, fresh (1 pepper/74g) 20 cals	0	3
Peppers: sweet, red, fresh (1 pepper/74g) 20 cals	0	5
Potato chips: fast-food type, fried in beef tallow (1 regular order/ 76g) 237 cals	58	5
Potato chips: fast-food type, fried in vegetable oil (1 regular order/ 76g) 235 cals	30	5
Potato chips: frozen oven-ready chips, heated in oven (10 chips/ 50g) 111 cals	21	3
Potato chips: restaurant type (par-fried then frozen and finished in vegetable oil) (10 chips/50g) 158 cals	20	3

	RiskPoints ✗	LifePoints ✔
Potato crisps: *see* Crisps in the 'Snacks and Sweets' section of the Drinks, Desserts, Snacks and Sauces group		
Potato dishes: au gratin, made with butter (1 cup/245g) 323 cals	104	14
Potato dishes: baked potato topped with baked beans (1 potato/310g) 338 cals	1	20
Potato dishes: baked potato topped with baked beans and margarine (1 potato/315g) 372 cals	11	20
Potato dishes: baked potato topped with butter (1 potato/290g) 256 cals	19	12
Potato dishes: baked potato topped with cheddar cheese and butter (1 potato/330g) 370 cals	61	19
Potato dishes: baked potato topped with cheese sauce (1 potato/296g) 474 cals	124	18
Potato dishes: baked potato topped with cheese sauce and bacon (1 potato/299g) 451 cals	115	21
Potato dishes: baked potato topped with cheese sauce and broccoli (1 potato/339g) 403 cals	96	23
Potato dishes: baked potato topped with cheese sauce and chilli (1 potato/395g) 482 cals	119	28
Potato dishes: baked potato topped with coleslaw (1 potato/290g) 262 cals	4	14

	RiskPoints ✗	LifePoints ✔
Potato dishes: baked potato topped with cottage cheese (1 potato/310g) 322 cals	10	21
Potato dishes: baked potato topped with margarine (1 potato/290g) 254 cals	9	12
Potato dishes: baked potato topped with sour cream and chives (1 potato/302g) 393 cals	56	16
Potato dishes: hashed browns (½ cup/72g) 151 cals	32	3
Potato dishes: mashed, made from instant granules with milk, water and margarine added (1 cup/210g) 166 cals	11	7
Potato dishes: mashed, made with whole milk and margarine (1 cup/210g) 223 cals	22	8
Potato dishes: mashed, made with whole milk, no margarine (1 cup/210g) 162 cals	6	9
Potato dishes: O'Brien, made with milk, onion, breadcrumbs and butter (1 cup/194g) 157 cals	13	8
Potato dishes: scalloped, made with butter (1 cup/245g) 211 cals	50	12
Potato flour: (1 cup/179g) 628 cals	3	29
Potato pancakes: (1 pancake/76g) 207 cals	28	7
Potato salad: (½ cup/125g) 179 cals	25	4
Potatoes: baked, flesh and skin (1 medium potato/202g) 220 cals	0	12

	RiskPoints ✗	LifePoints ✔
Potatoes: baked, flesh only (flesh from 1 medium potato/156g) 145 cals	0	7
Potatoes: baked, skin only (skin from 1 medium potato/58g) 115 cals	0	7
Potatoes: boiled, flesh only (flesh from 1 medium potato/136g) 118 cals	0	6
Potatoes: boiled, skin only (skin from 1 medium potato/34g) 27 cals	0	2
Potatoes: canned (1 small potato/ 35g) 21 cals	0	1
Potatoes: microwaved, flesh and skin (1 medium potato/202g) 212 cals	0	11
Pumpkin: boiled (½ cup mashed/ 122g) 24 cals	0	3
Pumpkin: canned (½ cup/122g) 41 cals	1	10
Radicchio: fresh (1 cup shredded/ 40g) 9 cals	0	1
Radishes: fresh (½ cup slices/ 58g) 10 cals	0	1
Radishes: oriental, fresh (½ cup slices/44g) 8 cals	0	1
Ratatouille: homemade (½ cup/ 107g) 133 cals	30	3
Runner beans: see 'Green beans'		
Salad: mixed vegetable, without dressing (1½ cups/207g) 33 cals	0	9
Salad: mixed vegetable without dressing, with cheese and egg (1½ cups/217g) 102 cals	22	11

	RiskPoints ✗	LifePoints ✔
Salad: mixed vegetable without dressing, with shrimp (1½ cups/236g) 106 cals	6	19
Salsify: boiled (½ cup slices/68g) 46 cals	0	3
Sandwich spread: with chopped pickle (1 tbsp/15g) 60 cals	13	0
Sauerkraut: canned, solids and liquid (1 cup/236g) 45 cals	0	9
Shallots: fresh (1 tbsp chopped/10g) 7 cals	0	0
Spinach: boiled (1 cup/180g) 41 cals	1	25
Spinach: canned, drained solids (1 cup/214g) 49 cals	2	22
Spinach: fresh (1 cup chopped/56g) 12 cals	0	10
Spinach: frozen, chopped or leaf, boiled (1 cup/190g) 53 cals	0	22
Spinach soufflé (1 cup/136g) 219 cals	53	18
Spring greens: see 'Cabbage, savoy'		
Squash: summer varieties, boiled (1 cup slices/180g) 36 cals	1	6
Squash: winter varieties, baked (1 cup cubes/205g) 80 cals	3	10
String beans: see 'Green beans'		
Swede: boiled (½ cup cubes/85g) 33 cals	0	3
Swede: fresh (½ cup cubes/70g) 25 cals	0	3
Sweetcorn: see Corn, sweet		
Sweet potatoes: baked in skin (½ sweet potato/57g) 59 cals	0	6

	RiskPoints ✗	LifePoints ✔
Sweet potatoes: boiled without skin (¼ cup mashed/82g) 86 cals	0	7
Tomato juice: (6 fl oz/182g) 31 cals	0	6
Tomato paste: canned (½ cup/ 131g) 110 cals	2	15
Tomato purée: canned (½ cup/ 125g) 51 cals	0	6
Tomato sauce: canned (½ cup/ 122g) 37 cals	0	5
Tomato soup: condensed and made with equal amount of milk (1 cup/8 fl oz/248g) 161 cals	29	11
Tomato soup: condensed and made with equal amount of water (1 cup/8 fl oz/244g) 85 cals	4	5
Tomato soup: dehydrated then made with water (1 pkt/6 fl oz/ 199g) 78 cals	8	2
Tomatoes: red, boiled (1 cup/ 240g) 65 cals	2	8
Tomatoes: red, canned (1 cup/ 240g) 48 cals	1	7
Tomatoes: red, fresh (1 tomato/ 123g) 26 cals	1	3
Tomatoes: sun-dried (8 pieces/ 16g) 41 cals	1	4
Tomatoes: sun-dried, packed in oil, drained (7 pieces/21g) 45 cals	7	2
Turnip greens: boiled (1 cup chopped/144g) 29 cals	0	16
Turnip greens: fresh (1 cup chopped/55g) 15 cals	0	10
Turnips: boiled (½ cup mashed/ 115g) 21 cals	0	2

	RiskPoints ✗	LifePoints ✔
Turnips: fresh (½ cup cubes/65g) 18 cals	0	2
Vegetable juice cocktail: canned (6 fl oz/182g) 35 cals	0	7
Vegetable soup: canned, chunky, ready-to-serve (1 cup/8 fl oz/ 240g) 122 cals	9	8
Vegetables: mixed, canned, drained solids (1 cup/163g) 77 cals	1	10
Vegetables: mixed, frozen pack, then boiled (1 cup/182g) 107 cals	0	11
Water chestnuts: Chinese, canned, solids and liquid (½ cup slices/ 70g) 35 cals	0	1
Watercress: fresh (½ cup chopped/17g) 2 cals	0	1
Yams: boiled or baked (½ cup cubes/68g) 79 cals	0	3
Yeast extract: fortified with vitamin B12 (1 tsp/5g) 9 cals	0	11
Yellow beans: boiled (1 cup/ 125g) 44 cals	0	6

GROUP FOUR: LEGUMES, NUTS AND SEEDS

Legumes and Beans

	RiskPoints ✗	LifePoints ✓
Adzuki beans: boiled (½ cup/ 115g) 147 cals	0	13
Baked beans: normal (i.e. vegetarian) (½ cup/127g) 118 cals	1	8
Baked beans: on toast (½ can beans and 1 slice toast with butter/233g) 263 cals	4	17
Baked beans: on toast (½ can beans and 1 slice toast with butter/238g) 298 cals	22	17
Baked beans: with sausages (½ cup/128g) 182 cals	22	9
Black or turtle bean soup: (½ cup/4 fl oz/120g) 109 cals	0	9
Black or turtle beans: boiled (½ cup/86g) 114 cals	1	11
Black-eyed beans: boiled (½ cup/ 86g) 100 cals	1	13
Black-eyed beans: canned (½ cup/120g) 92 cals	1	7
Broadbeans: boiled (½ cup/85g) 94 cals	0	9
Broadbeans: canned (½ cup/ 128g) 91 cals	0	6
Broadbeans: raw (½ cup/75g) 256 cals	2	25
Cannellini beans: boiled (½ cup/ 90g) 128 cals	1	12
Cannellini beans: canned (½ cup/ 131g) 153 cals	0	12
Chick peas: boiled (½ cup/82g) 134 cals	5	12

	RiskPoints ✗	LifePoints ✔
Chick peas: brown, boiled (½ cup/77g) 85 cals	2	9
Chick peas: canned (½ cup/ 120g) 143 cals	3	11
Green beans: *See* Vegetables and Vegetable Products group		
Haricot beans: boiled (½ cup/ 91g) 129 cals	1	12
Haricot beans: canned (½ cup/ 131g) 148 cals	1	12
Haricot beans: sprouted, boiled (½ cup/85g) 66 cals	1	12
Kidney beans: boiled (½ cup/ 88g) 112 cals	1	12
Kidney beans: canned (½ cup/ 128g) 104 cals	0	8
Lentils: boiled (½ cup/99g) 115 cals	0	16
Lentils: sprouted, raw (½ cup/ 38g) 40 cals	0	5
Lentils: sprouted, stir-fried (½ cup/38g) 38 cals	0	4
Lima beans: boiled (½ cup/85g) 105 cals	0	6
Mung beans: boiled (½ cup/ 101g) 106 cals	0	13
Mung beans: sprouted, boiled (1 cup/124g) 26 cals	0	5
Mung beans: sprouted, boiled (½ cup/62g) 13 cals	0	2
Mung beans: sprouted, canned, drained solids (½ cup/62g) 7 cals	0	1
Peanuts: *see* 'Nuts and Nut Products'		

	RiskPoints ✗	LifePoints ✔
Peas: split, boiled (½ cup/98g) 116 cals	0	9
Pinto beans: boiled (½ cup/85g) 116 cals	1	14
Pinto beans: canned (½ cup/ 120g) 94 cals	0	9
Refried beans: canned (½ cup/ 126g) 135 cals	3	12
Soya beans: boiled (½ cup/86g) 149 cals	19	12
Soya beans: sprouted, raw (½ cup/35g) 43 cals	5	6
Soya beans: sprouted, steamed (½ cup/47g) 38 cals	5	4
Soya beans: sprouted, stir-fried (½ cup/47g) 59 cals	8	7

Legume and Bean Products

	RiskPoints ✗	LifePoints ✔
Bacon: meatless (1 strip/8g) 25 cals	5	3
Bean pâté: made with lentils (1 serving/75g) 79 cals	0	11
Burrito: with beans (2 burritos/ 217g) 447 cals	51	28
Carob bar: (1 bar/87g) 464 cals	71	17
Chilli with beans: canned (½ cup 128g) 143 cals	22	10
Dhal: made with mung beans (1 serving/235g) 130 cals	23	13
Falafel: (1 patty/17g) 57 cals	7	2
Hummus: (½ cup/123g) 210 cals	25	12

	RiskPoints ✗	LifePoints ✔
Meat substitute: textured vegetable protein (TVP) (1oz/28g) 88 cals	2	21
Miso: (1 tbsp/17g) 35 cals	2	2
Natto: (½ cup/88g) 187 cals	24	13
Sausage: meatless (1 link/25g) 64 cals	11	9
Soya milk: (1 cup/240g) 79 cals	11	7
Soya sauce: (1 tbsp/18g) 10 cals	0	1
Soya bean oil: *see* 'Margarines, Oils and Spreads' in the Drinks, Desserts, Snacks and Sauces group		
Tempeh: (½ cup/83g) 165 cals	15	14
Tofu: fried (1 piece/13g) 35 cals	6	1
Tofu: raw firm (¼ block/81g) 117 cals	17	12
Tofu: raw regular (¼ block/116g) 88 cals	13	8

Nuts and Nut Products

	RiskPoints ✗	LifePoints ✔
Almond butter: (1 tbsp/16g) 101 cals	23	3
Almond oil: *see* 'Margarines, Oils and Spreads' in the Drinks, Desserts, Snacks and Sauces group		
Almonds: dried, blanched (24 kernels/28g) 166 cals	37	5
Almonds: dry roasted, unblanched (24 kernels/28g) 167 cals	36	6
Almonds: ground (1oz/28g) 168 cals	36	5

	RiskPoints ✗	LifePoints ✔
Almonds: oil roasted, unblanched (22 kernels/28.4g) 176 cals	40	7
Brazil nuts: dried (6–8 kernels/ 28.4g) 186 cals	47	5
Cashews: dry roasted (1oz/28.4g) 163 cals	32	5
Cashews: nut butter, plain (1 tbsp/16g) 94 cals	19	2
Cashews: oil roasted (1oz/28.4g) 164 cals	34	5
Chestnuts: sweet, boiled and steamed (1oz/28.4g) 37 cals	0	2
Chestnuts: sweet, roasted (1oz/ 28.4g) 70 cals	1	3
Coconut: cream, canned (liquid expressed from grated meat) (1 tbsp/19g) 36 cals	22	0
Coconut: creamed (1oz/28.4g) 194 cals	130	2
Coconut: meat, dried (desiccated) not sweetened (1oz/28.4g) 187 cals	121	2
Coconut: meat, raw (1 cup shredded or grated/80g) 283 cals	178	5
Filberts or hazelnuts: dried, unblanched (1oz/28.4g) 179 cals	44	5
Filberts or hazelnuts: dry roasted, unblanched (1oz/28.4g) 188 cals	47	5
Filberts or hazelnuts: oil roasted, unblanched (1oz/28.4g) 187 cals	45	5
Ginkgo nuts: dried (1oz/28.4g) 99 cals	1	6
Ginkgo nuts: raw (1oz/28.4g) 52 cals	1	3

	RiskPoints ✗	LifePoints ✓
Hazelnut oil: *see* 'Margarines, Oils and Spreads' in the Drinks, Desserts, Snacks and Sauces group		
Macadamia nuts: dried (1oz/ 28.4g) 199 cals	52	3
Macadamia nuts: oil roasted (10– 12 kernels/28.4g) 204 cals	54	2
Mixed nuts with peanuts: dry roasted (10–12 kernels/28.4g) 169 cals	36	5
Mixed nuts with peanuts: oil roasted (1oz/28.4g) 175 cals	39	6
Peanut butter: chunk style (2 tbsp/32g) 188 cals	39	7
Peanut butter: smooth style (2 tbsp/32g) 188 cals	39	6
Peanuts: boiled (½ cup/32g) 102 cals	17	4
Peanuts: dry roasted (1oz/28g) 164 cals	34	7
Peanuts: oil roasted (1oz/28g) 163 cals	34	8
Peanuts: raw (1oz/28g) 159 cals	34	10
Pecans: dried (1oz/28.4g) 189 cals	48	4
Pecans: dry roasted (20 halves/ 28.4g) 187 cals	45	3
Pecans: oil roasted (20 halves/ 28.4g) 195 cals	50	3
Pine nuts: dried (15 kernels/ 28.4g) 146 cals	35	6
Pistachio: dried (47 kernels/ 28.4g) 164 cals	34	6
Pistachio: dry roasted (47 kernels/28.4g) 172 cals	37	4

	RiskPoints ✗	LifePoints ✔
Pumpkin and squash: seed kernels, dried (142 kernels/ 28.4g) 154 cals	32	7
Pumpkin and squash: seed kernels, roasted (142 kernels/ 28.4g) 148 cals	29	7
Sesame oil: *see* 'Margarines, Oils and Spreads' in the Drinks, Desserts, Snacks and Sauces group		
Sesame: seed butter paste (1 tbsp/ 169) 95 cals	20	6
Sesame: seeds, whole roasted and toasted (1 tbsp/9g) 51 cals	10	4
Sunflower oil: *see* 'Margarines, Oils and Spreads' in the Drinks, Desserts, Snacks and Sauces group		
Sunflower: seed butter (1 tbsp/ 69g) 93 cals	19	5
Sunflower: seed kernels, dried (1oz/28.4g) 162 cals	35	13
Sunflower: seed kernels, dry roasted (1oz/28.4g) 165 cals	35	9
Sunflower: seed kernels, oil roasted (1oz/28.4g) 175 cals	40	9
Tahini: made from roasted and toasted sesame kernels, the most common type (1 tbsp/15g) 89 cals	20	5
Walnut oil: *see* 'Margarines, Oils and Spreads' in the Drinks, Desserts, Snacks and Sauces group		
Walnuts: dried (1oz/28.4g) 182 cals	43	4

GROUP FIVE: MEAT, FISH AND DAIRY

MEAT
Beef

	RiskPoints ✗	LifePoints ✔
Beef cured pastrami: (2 slices/56g) 198 cals	44	10
Beef dripping: (1 tbsp/13g) 115 cals	47	0
Beef jerky: chopped and pressed (1oz/28g) 96 cals	12	12
Beerwurst (beer salami): *see* Sausages and Luncheon Meats		
Bologna: *see* Sausages and Luncheon Meats		
Brisket: lean and fat, braised (3oz/85g) 327 cals	78	18
Brisket: lean only, braised (3oz/85g) 206 cals	29	21
Chilli con carne: (1 cup/253g) 256 cals	25	25
Corned beef: jellied loaf (2 slices/56g) 87 cals	11	8
Cured thin-sliced beef: (1oz/28g) 50 cals	3	7
Frankfurter: beef (1 frankfurter 57g) 180 cals	51	7
Hotdog: in roll (1 link in roll/141g) 365 cals	42	18
Hotdog: plain (1 hotdog link/98g) 242 cals	38	13
Meat-based snack sticks: smoked (1 stick/20g) 109 cals	30	3
Mince: regular, baked, medium (3oz/85g) 244 cals	52	18

	RiskPoints ✗	LifePoints ✔
Mince: regular, grilled, medium (3oz/85g) 246 cals	51	19
Mince: regular, pan-fried, medium (3oz/85g) 260 cals	56	19
Porterhouse steak: lean and fat, grilled (3oz/85g) 259 cals	56	19
Rib steak: lean and fat, grilled (3oz/85g) 275 cals	65	18
Rump steak: lean and fat, grilled (3oz/85g) 190 cals	26	20
Sirloin steak: lean and fat, grilled (3oz/85g) 208 cals	35	21
Soup: beef and noodles, canned (1 cup/8fl oz/244g) 83 cals	17	5
Soup: beef and tomato with noodles (1 cup/8 fl oz/244g) 139 cals	23	5
Soup: beef and vegetable (1 cup/ 8 fl oz/244g) 78 cals	6	5
Soup: beef broth, bouillon and consommé (1 cup/8 fl oz/241g) 29 cals	0	2
Soup: oxtail (1 cup/8 fl oz/253g) 71 cals	9	2
Steak and kidney pie: (1 serving 250g) 808 cals	166	25
Stew: beef, homemade (1 cup 252g) 222 cals	13	22
Stroganoff: (1 serving/349g) 603 cals	150	35
T-bone steak: lean and fat, grilled (3oz/85g) 253 cals	54	19
Tenderloin: lean and fat, grilled (3oz/85g) 247 cals	50	20

	RiskPoints ✗	LifePoints ✔
Tenderloin: lean and fat, roasted (3oz/85g) 282 cals	64	18

Chicken

	RiskPoints ✗	LifePoints ✔
Breast meat and skin: fried in batter (3oz/85g) 221 cals	28	13
Breast meat and skin: roasted (3oz/85g) 167 cals	16	15
Breast meat and skin: stewed (3oz/85g) 156 cals	15	10
Chicken fat: (1 tbsp/12g) 115 cals	31	0
Chicken meat: canned, boned with stock (½ can/71g) 117 cals	14	8
Chicken roll: light meat (1 slice/1oz/28g) 45 cals	5	2
Chicken salad spread: (1 tbsp/13g) 26 cals	4	0
Chicken spread: canned (1 tbsp/13g) 25 cals	3	1
Chicken stock cubes: dry (1 cube/5g) 10 cals	0	0
Drumstick meat and skin: fried in batter (1 drumstick/72g) 193 cals	28	9
Drumstick meat and skin: roasted (1 drumstick/52g) 112 cals	14	7
Fast food: boneless pieces, breaded and fried, plain (6 pieces/102g) 290 cals	44	12
Fast food: breast or wing, light meat, breaded and fried (2 pieces/163g) 494 cals	73	22

	RiskPoints ✗	LifePoints ✔
Fast food: drumstick or thigh, dark meat, breaded and fried (2 pieces/148g) 431 cals	66	20
Frankfurter: chicken (1 frankfurter/45g) 116 cals	21	4
Salad: chicken and vegetable, with dressing (1½ cups/263g) 280 cals	43	16
Salad: chicken and vegetable, without dressing (1½ cups/218g) 105 cals	5	15
Soup: chicken and mushroom (1 cup/8 fl oz/244g) 132 cals	22	4
Soup: chicken and vegetable (1 cup/8 fl oz/240g) 166 cals	12	9
Soup: chicken noodle, canned chunky, ready-to-serve (1 cup/8 fl oz/240g) 175 cals	15	9
Soup: cream of chicken (1 cup/8 fl oz/248g) 191 cals	34	9
Sweet and sour chicken (1 serving/453g) 626 cals	41	25
Wing meat and skin: fried in batter (1 wing/49g) 159 cals	26	5
Wing meat and skin: roasted (1 wing/34g) 99 cals	16	4

Goose

	RiskPoints ✗	LifePoints ✔
Meat and skin: roasted (3oz/85g) 259 cals	46	12
Meat only: roasted (3oz/85g) 202 cals	29	15

	RiskPoints ✗	LifePoints ✔
Pâté de foie gras (goose liver pâté): smoked (1oz/28g) 131 cals	31	11

Gravy

	RiskPoints ✗	LifePoints ✔
Au jus: (½ cup/119) 19 cals	0	3
Beef: (½ cup/116g) 61 cals	10	3
Brown: dehydrated then prepared with water (½ cup/129g) 37 cals	3	1
Chicken: (½ cup/119g) 94 cals	16	2
Turkey: (½ cup/118g) 60 cals	6	3

Lamb

	RiskPoints ✗	LifePoints ✔
Chop: lean and fat, grilled (3oz/85g) 307 cals	80	19
Chop: lean and fat, roasted (3oz/85g) 305 cals	81	18
Leg: lean and fat, roasted (3oz/85g) 219 cals	43	20
Moussaka: (1 serving/225g) 439 cals	79	24
Scotch broth: (1 cup/8 fl oz/241g) 80 cals	16	5
Shepherd's pie: (1 serving/225g) 268 cals	42	21

Pork

	RiskPoints ✗	LifePoints ✔
Bacon: back, grilled (3oz/85g) 157 cals	18	18

	RiskPoints ✗	LifePoints ✔
Bacon: gammon, grilled pan-fried or roasted (3oz/85g) 490 cals	111	22
Bacon: meatless (i.e. vegetarian): *see* 'Legume and Bean Products' in the Legumes, Nuts and Seeds group.		
Bacon: streaky, grilled, pan-fried or roasted (3oz/85g) 390 cals	81	24
Chop: lean and fat, braised (3oz/85g) 213 cals	37	15
Chop: lean and fat, grilled (3oz/85g) 224 cals	36	20
Chop: lean and fat, pan-fried (3oz/85g) 225 cals	40	17
Chop: lean and fat, roasted (3oz/85g) 217 cals	37	17
Ham patties: grilled (1 patty/59g) 203 cals	49	7
Ham, cured: chopped, canned (1 slice/21g) 50 cals	9	3
Ham, cured: croquettes, grilled (1 croquette/59g) 203 cals	49	7
Ham, cured: lean and fat, roasted (3oz/85g) 207 cals	38	14
Headcheese: pork (1 slice or 1oz/28g) 60 cals	11	3
Lard: (1 tbsp/12g) 115 cals	37	0
Leg: lean and fat, roasted (3oz/85g) 232 cals	41	17
Liver: braised (3oz/85g) 140 cals	9	45
Liver sausage: *see* 'Sausages and Luncheon Meats'		
Liverwurst: *see* 'Sausages and Luncheon Meats'		

	RiskPoints ✗	LifePoints ✔
Loin: lean and fat, braised (3oz/85g) 203 cals	32	15
Loin: lean and fat, grilled (3oz/85g) 206 cals	33	18
Loin: lean and fat, roasted (3oz/85g) 211 cals	34	19
Minced: cooked (3oz/85g) 252 cals	49	16
Pork pies: (1 individual pie/210g) 730 cals	121	34
Pork scratchings: (1oz/28g) 155 cals	24	4
Sausage: fresh, cooked without additional fat (1 sausage/27g) 100 cals	21	6
Sausage roll: (1 roll/55g) 263 cals	58	2
Shoulder: lean and fat, roasted (3oz/85g) 248 cals	50	16
Soup: ham and split pea, canned, chunky ready-to-serve (1 cup/8 fl oz/240g) 185 cals	11	10
Spare ribs: lean and fat, braised (3oz/85g) 337 cals	70	19
Trotters: pickled pig's feet (1oz/28g) 58 cals	11	2

Rabbit

	RiskPoints ✗	LifePoints ✔
All cuts: roasted (3oz/85g) 167 cals	17	21
All cuts: stewed (3oz/85g) 175 cals	17	20

Sausages and Luncheon Meats

	RiskPoints ✗	LifePoints ✔
Beef luncheon meat: loaved (1 slice/28g) 87 cals	23	7
Beerwurst (beer salami): pork (1 slice/23g) 76 cals	22	3
Berliner: (1 slice/23g) 53 cals	10	4
Blood sausage or blood pudding: (1 slice/25g) 95 cals	25	3
Bockwurst: (1: link/65g) 200 cals	49	9
Bologna: beef (1 slice or 1oz/28g) 88 cals	25	3
Bologna: beef and pork (1 slice/23g) 73 cals	18	3
Bologna: pork (1 slice/23g) 57 cals	11	3
Braunschweiger (liver sausage): smoked (1 slice/18g) 65 cals	14	12
Bratwurst: (1 link/70g) 226 cals	52	12
Chicken liver pâté: canned (1 tbsp/13g) 26 cals	4	9
Chorizo: (1 link/60g) 273 cals	64	15
Cured ham: minced and pressed (1 slice/21g) 55 cals	11	3
Goose liver pâté: see 'Pâté de foie gras'		
Ham and cheese spread: (1 tbsp/15g) 37 cals	9	2
Ham salad spread: (1 tbsp/15g) 32 cals	5	1
Ham: chopped, spiced, canned (1 slice/21g) 50 cals	9	3
Headcheese: see 'Pork'		

	RiskPoints ✗	LifePoints ✓
Italian sausage: cooked (1 link/67g) 216 cals	45	13
Liver sausage (liverwurst): pork (1 slice/18g) 59 cals	14	11
Mixed pork and beef sausage: cooked (1 link/13g) 51 cals	12	1
Mortadella: (1 slice/15g) 47 cals	10	2
Pâté de foie gras: canned, smoked (1 tbsp/13g) 60 cals	14	6
Pâté: mixed meat or meat not specified (1 tbsp/13g) 41 cals	9	3
Pepperoni: (1 slice/5g) 27 cals	6	1
Polish-style sausage: (1 sausage/227g) 740 cals	175	33
Pork links: cooked (1 link/13g) 48 cals	10	2
Pork luncheon meat: canned (1 slice/21g) 70 cals	16	2
Sandwich spread: pork and beef (1 tbsp/15g) 35 cals	6	1
Sausage meat: cooked (1oz/28g) 103 cals	22	6
Smoked link sausage: pork, grilled (1 link/68g) 265 cals	57	15
Thuringer: (1 slice/23g) 77 cals	20	7
Turkey and ham luncheon meat: (1 slice/28g) 36 cals	3	3
Vienna sausage: canned (1 sausage 16g) 45 cals	11	1

Turkey

	RiskPoints ✗	LifePoints ✔
Boneless turkey meat: roasted (3oz/85g) 132 cals	12	15
Breast: meat and skin, roasted (3oz/85g) 161 cals	15	12
Dark meat: roasted (3oz/85g) 159 cals	25	13
Leg: meat and skin, roasted (3oz/85g) 177 cals	20	13
Light meat: roasted (3oz/85g) 133 cals	6	13
Mince turkey: cooked (1 patty/82g) 193 cals	26	11
Soup: turkey, canned, chunky, ready-to-serve (1 cup/8 fl oz/236g) 135 cals	11	16
Turkey meat: canned with stock (3oz/85g) 139 cals	14	11
Turkey patties: breaded, battered and fried (1 patty/3oz/85g) 266 cals	42	9
Turkey roll: made from light and dark meat (3oz/85g) 127 cals	14	10
Turkey sticks: breaded, battered and fried (1 stick/2¼oz/64g) 179 cals	27	6

Venison

	RiskPoints ✗	LifePoints ✔
Roasted: (3oz/85g) 134 cals	7	14

FISH AND SEAFOOD

NOTE: throughout this section, 'moist heat' includes cooking methods such as steaming, stewing and inclusion in soups and sauces. 'Dry heat' includes methods such as grilling and baking.

	RiskPoints ✗	LifePoints ✔
Anchovy: canned in oil, drained solids (5 anchovies/20g) 42 cals	4	5
Bass: freshwater, cooked dry heat (1 fillet/62g) 91 cals	7	11
Carp: cooked dry heat (1 fillet/170g) 275 cals	30	25
Catfish: breaded and fried (1 fillet/87g) 199 cals	28	13
Caviar: black and red granular (1 tbsp/16g) 40 cals	7	11
Clam: breaded and fried (10 small clams/94g) 190 cals	26	22
Clam: cooked moist heat (10 small clams/94g) 139 cals	4	28
Cod liver oil: (1 tbsp/13g) 123 cals	34	0
Cod: cooked dry heat (1 fillet/180g) 189 cals	3	22
Cod: dried and salted (3oz/85g) 247 cals	5	29
Crab cakes: (1 cake/60g) 93 cals	11	15
Crab: cooked moist heat (3oz/85g) 87 cals	3	19
Eel: cooked dry heat (1 fillet/159g) 375 cals	59	24
Fish and chips: 1 fillet plaice fried in batter and 1 regular order of chips fried in vegetable oil (256g) 737 cals	111	19

	RiskPoints ✗	LifePoints ✔
Fish fillet: battered or breaded and fried (1 fillet/91g) 211 cals	27	12
Fish fingers: (1 finger/28g) 76 cals	8	4
Fish pie: (1 serving/200g) 256 cals	36	17
Flatfish (flounder and sole species): cooked dry heat (1 fillet/127g) 149 cals	4	18
Gefiltefish: sweet recipe (1 piece/42g) 35 cals	1	3
Haddock: cooked dry heat (1 fillet/150g) 168 cals	3	23
Haddock: smoked (3oz/85g) 99 cals	2	14
Herring: kippered (1 fillet/40g) 87 cals	12	13
Herring: pickled (1 piece/15g) 39 cals	6	3
Kedgeree: (1 serving/115g) 174 cals	20	14
Kipper: see 'Herring'		
Lobster: cooked moist heat (3oz/85g) 83 cals	1	14
Lox: *see* 'Salmon'	0	0
Mackerel: cooked with dry heat (1 fillet/88g) 231 cals	39	20
Mussels: cooked moist heat (3oz/85g) 146 cals	9	24
Oyster stew: canned, condensed (1 cup/8 fl oz/246g) 118 cals	37	18
Oyster: breaded and fried (6 medium oysters/88g) 173 cals	27	23

	RiskPoints ✗	LifePoints ✔
Oyster: canned (3oz/85g) 59 cals	5	22
Perch: cooked dry heat (1 fillet/ 46g) 54 cals	1	8
Pickled herring: *see* 'Herring'		
Prawn: breaded and fried (4 large shrimp/30g) 73 cals	9	5
Prawn: canned (3oz/85g) 102 cals	4	11
Roe: cooked dry heat (3oz/85g) 173 cals	17	25
Salad: seafood, vegetable and pasta, without dressing (1½ cups/ 417g) 379 cals	52	24
Salad: tuna (3oz/85g) 159 cals	19	11
Salmon: canned, drained solids with bone (3oz/85g) 130 cals	15	11
Salmon: cooked dry heat (½ fillet/ 155g) 335 cals	42	26
Salmon: smoked (lox), regular (3oz/85g) 99 cals	9	14
Salmon: wild, cooked dry heat (½ fillet/154g) 280 cals	31	39
Sardine: canned in oil, drained solids with bone (2 sardines/24g) 50 cals	6	11
Sardine: canned in oil, drained solids with bone (1 can/92g) 191 cals	26	22
Sardine: canned in tomato sauce, drained solids with bone (2 sardines/76g) 135 cals	22	17
Sardine: canned in tomato sauce, drained solids with bone (1 can/ 370g) 659 cals	110	51

	RiskPoints ✗	LifePoints ✔
Scallop: breaded and fried (2 large scallops/31g) 67 cals	8	3
Scampi: breaded and fried (6 pieces/164g) 454 cals	62	16
Sole: *see* Flatfish		
Trout: cooked dry heat (1 fillet 62g) 118 cals	13	17
Tuna: canned in oil, drained solids (3oz/85g) 168 cals	17	19
Tuna: canned in water, drained solids (3oz/85g) 99 cals	1	20
Whitefish: cooked dry heat (1 fillet/154g) 265 cals	28	23
Whitefish: smoked (3oz/85g) 92 cals	1	15
Whiting: cooked dry heat (1 fillet/ 72g) 83 cals	3	13

DAIRY
Butter

	RiskPoints ✗	LifePoints ✔
Butter (1 pat/5g) 36 cals	18	0
Ghee: anhydrous butter oil (1 tbsp/13g) 112 cals	46	0

Cheese

	RiskPoints ✗	LifePoints ✔
Brie: (1oz/28g) 93 cals	36	5
Camembert: (1oz/28g) 84 cals	32	5
Cheddar: (1oz/28g) 114 cals	42	5
Cheese and ham spread: *see* 'Sausages and Luncheon Meats'		

	RiskPoints ✗	LifePoints ✔
Cheese fondue: (1 serving/80g) 229 cals	77	12
Cheese soufflé: (1 cup/136g) 343 cals	86	16
Cheshire: (1oz/28g) 108 cals	40	5
Cottage: creamed, large or small curd (4oz/113g) 117 cals	24	8
Cottage: low-fat 2% fat (4oz/113g) 101 cals	10	9
Cream cheese: (1oz/28g) 98 cals	46	1
Edam: (1oz/28g) 100 cals	36	6
Feta: (1oz/28g) 74 cals	31	7
Goat: hard type (1oz/28g) 128 cals	52	7
Goat: semi-soft type (1oz/28g) 103 cals	43	3
Goat: soft type (1oz/28g) 76 cals	30	3
Gouda: (1oz/28g) 100 cals	36	6
Gruyere: (1oz/28g) 116 cals	39	7
Mozzarella: part-skimmed milk (1oz/28g) 71 cals	21	4
Mozzarella: whole milk (1oz/28g) 79 cals	27	3
Parmesan: grated (1oz/28g) 128 cals	40	8
Parmesan: grated (1 tbsp/5g) 23 cals	7	1
Processed: (1oz/28g) 93 cals	32	5
Ricotta: whole milk (¼ cup/62g) 108 cals	38	5
Roquefort: (1oz/28g) 103 cals	40	5
Swiss: (1oz/28g) 105 cals	37	7
Welsh rarebit: (1 serving/60g) 219 cals	62	8

Cream

	RiskPoints ✗	LifePoints ✔
Cream: double (1 tbsp/15g) 37 cals	17	0
Cream: single (1 tbsp/15g) 29 cals	13	0
Cream substitute: non-dairy powder (1 tsp/2g) 11 cals	4	0
Dessert topping: non-dairy, pressurized (1 tbsp/4g) 11 cals	5	0
Sour cream: (1 tbsp/12g) 26 cals	11	0
Whipped cream topping: pressurized (1 tbsp/3g) 8 cals	3	0
Whipping cream: heavy (1 tbsp/15g) 52 cals	25	0
Whipping cream: light (1 tbsp/15g) 44 cals	21	0

Eggs: Chicken

	RiskPoints ✗	LifePoints ✔
Dried (1 tbsp/5g) 30 cals	5	3
Egg custard: baked (½ cup/14g) 148 cals	24	8
Egg substitute: powder (0.35oz/9g) 44 cals	3	4
Fried: (1 large egg/46g) 92 cals	17	6
Hard-boiled: (1 large egg/50g) 78 cals	13	7
Omelette: (2 eggs/120g) 182 cals	34	12
Poached: (1 large egg/50g) 75 cals	12	6
Quiche Lorraine: (1 serving/115g) 450 cals	107	15

	RiskPoints ✗	LifePoints ✔
Raw: white only (1 large egg white/33g) 17 cals	0	1
Raw: yolk only (1 large egg yolk/16g) 59 cals	12	5
Raw: yolk and white (1 large egg/50g) 75 cals	12	7
Scotch egg: (1 egg/115g) 321 cals	67	13
Scrambled: (1 egg/60g) 100 cals	18	7

Eggs: Duck

	RiskPoints ✗	LifePoints ✔
Raw: (1 egg/70g) 130 cals	24	17

Eggs: Goose

	RiskPoints ✗	LifePoints ✔
Raw: (1 egg/144g) 267 cals	47	27

Eggs: Quail

	RiskPoints ✗	LifePoints ✔
Raw: (1 egg/9g) 14 cals	2	1

Milk: Cow's

	RiskPoints ✗	LifePoints ✔
Buttermilk: cultured from skimmed milk (1 cup/245g) 99 cals	10	10
Buttermilk: dried (1 tbsp/6g) 25 cals	1	3
Condensed milk: canned, sweetened (1 fl oz/38g) 123 cals	15	3

223

	RiskPoints ✗	LifePoints ✔
Dried skimmed milk: non-fat solids (¼ cup/30g) 109 cals	1	15
Dried whole milk: (¼ cup/32g) 159 cals	40	12
Evaporated: canned, unsweetened (1 fl oz/31g) 42 cals	10	2
Malted milk beverage (1 cup milk + ¾ oz pwd/265g) 236 cals	44	17
Whole milk: (1 cup/244g) 157 cals	41	12
Semi-skimmed milk: (1 cup/244g) 136 cals	22	14
Skimmed milk: (1 cup/245g) 86 cals	2	12

Milk: Goat's

	RiskPoints ✗	LifePoints ✔
Goat's milk: (1 cup/244g) 168 cals	48	9

Milk: Sheep's

	RiskPoints ✗	LifePoints ✔
Ewe's milk: (1 cup/245g) 264 cals	84	22

Yogurt

	RiskPoints ✗	LifePoints ✔
Low-fat: (½ container/113g) 72 cals	8	8
Low-fat: with fruit (½ container/114g) 115 cals	5	7
Skimmed milk: (½ container/113g) 63 cals	0	9
Whole milk: (½ container/113g) 69 cals	17	5

GROUP SIX: DRINKS, DESSERTS, SNACKS AND SAUCES

Drinks

	RiskPoints ✗	LifePoints ✔
Apple juice: *see* Fruit and Fruit Juices group		
Apricot nectar: *see* Fruit and Fruit Juices group		
Capuccino: coffee made with cream and chocolate (1 cup/ 212g) 86 cals	33	1
Carbonated soft drink: e.g. lemonade (12 fl oz can/368g) 147 cals	0	0
Carrot juice: *see* the Vegetables and Vegetable Products group		
Cherry juice: *see* the Fruit and Fruit Juices group		
Cocoa: homemade from hot milk (1 cup/8 fl oz/250g) 218 cals	42	14
Coffee substitute: cereal grain beverage powder (1 tsp/2g) 9 cals	0	0
Coffee: brewed (1 cup/6 fl oz/ 177g) 4 cals	0	0
Coffee: instant decaffeinated powder (1 rounded tsp/2g) 4 cals	0	0
Coffee: instant regular powder (1 rounded tsp/2g) 4 cals	0	0
Cola: (12 fl oz can/370g) 152 cals	0	0
Cola: low-calorie (12 fl oz can/ 355g)	0	0
Cranberry juice: *see* the Fruit and Fruit Juices group		

	RiskPoints ✗	LifePoints ✓
Cranberry juice cocktail: *see* the Fruit and Fruit Juices group		
Eggnog: (½ cup/4 fl oz/127g) 171 cals	42	7
Ginger ale: (12 fl oz can/366g) 124 cals	0	0
Grape juice: *see* the Fruit and Fruit Juices group		
Grapefruit juice: *see* the Fruit and Fruit Juices group		
Lemon juice: *see* the Fruit and Fruit Juices group		
Lemonade: *see* 'Carbonated soft drink'		
Lime juice: *see* the Fruit and Fruit Juices group		
Malted milk: with added nutrients (1 cup/8 fl oz milk + 3 heaped tsp pwd/265g) 231 cals	40	34
Malted milk: with no added nutrients (1 cup/8 fl oz milk + 3 heaped tsp pwd/265g) 236 cals	44	17
Milkshake: chocolate (10 fl oz/ 283g) 359 cals	49	16
Milkshake: vanilla (10 fl oz/283g) 314 cals	39	14
Orange juice: *see* the Fruit and Fruit Juices group		
Passion-fruit juice: *see* the Fruit and Fruit Juices group		
Peach nectar: *see* the Fruit and Fruit Juices group		
Pear nectar: *see* the Fruit and Fruit Juices group		

	RiskPoints ✘	LifePoints ✔
Pineapple juice: *see* the Fruit and Fruit Juices group		
Prune juice: *see* the Fruit and Fruit Juices group		
Tea: herb (6 fl oz/178g) 2 cals	0	0
Tea: with milk (1 cup/8 fl oz/ 238g) 40cals	12	3
Tea: without milk (1 cup/6 fl oz/ 178g) 2 cals	0	0
Tomato juice: *see* the Vegetables and Vegetable Products group		
Tonic water: (12 fl oz can/366g) 124 cals	0	0
Vegetable juice cocktail: *see* the Vegetables and Vegetable Products group		
Vinegar: cider (1 tbsp/15g) 2 cals	0	0
Water: bottled mineral (1 cup/8 fl oz/237g)	0	0

Biscuits and Cookies

	RiskPoints ✘	LifePoints ✔
Brownie: (large brownie/56g) 227 cals	22	4
Chocolate chip cookie: soft-type (1 biscuit/15g) 69 cals	9	0
Chocolate wafers: (1 wafer/6g) 26 cals	2	0
Custard cream: (1 biscuit/14g) 72 cals	15	0
Digestive biscuit: chocolate-coated (large digestive/14g) 68 cals	11	1
Digestive biscuit: plain (large digestive/7g) 30 cals	1	0

	RiskPoints ✘	LifePoints ✔
Fig bars: (1 biscuit/16g) 56 cals	2	1
Fudge: cake-type (1 biscuit/21g) 73 cals	1	1
Ginger: (1 biscuit/7g) 29 cals	1	0
Peanut butter cookie: (1 biscuit/ 15g) 72 cals	8	1
Shortbread: plain (1 biscuit/8g) 40 cals	4	0

Cakes, Pastries and Puddings

As you can see, none of these can fairly be described as 'health food'! But if you really want to know the damage, here's the awful truth . . . !

	RiskPoints ✘	LifePoints ✔
Apple pie: (1 serving/155g) 411 cals	48	5
Apple strudel: (1 slice/71g) 195 cals	19	2
Bread and butter pudding: (1 serving/115g) 183 cals	34	6
Carrot cake: with cream cheese icing (1 serving/111g) 484 cals	73	6
Cheesecake: (1 serving/80g) 257 cals	69	4
Cherry pie: (1 serving/125g) 325 cals	34	2
Chocolate cake: with chocolate icing (1 serving/64g) 235 cals	26	3
Christmas pudding: (1 serving/ 115g) 350 cals	46	6
Coffee cake: crème-filling with chocolate icing (1 serving/90g) 298 cals	24	5

	RiskPoints ✗	LifePoints ✔
Cream puffs: (1 cream puff shell/ 66g) 239 cals	42	6
Danish pastry: (1 pastry/65g) 262 cals	36	7
Doughnuts: crème filling (1 doughnut/85g) 307 cals	52	7
Doughnuts: jam filling (1 doughnut/85g) 289 cals	39	6
Doughnuts: ring, glazed (1 medium doughnut/60g) 242 cals	34	6
Doughnuts: ring, plain (1 medium doughnut/47g) 198 cals	26	3
Eclairs: custard-filled with chocolate glaze (1 éclair/100g) 262 cals	39	7
Filo pastry: (1 sheet/19g) 57 cals	2	2
Fruit jelly: (½ cup/106g) 73 cals	0	1
Fruitcake: (1 small serving/43g) 139 cals	9	1
Gingerbread cake: (1 serving/ 74g) 263 cals	30	5
Ice cream cones: cake or wafer type (1 cone/4g) 17 cals	0	0
Icing: chocolate made with butter (1 serving/50g) 200 cals	26	0
Icing: chocolate made with margarine (1 serving/50g) 201 cals	14	0
Icing: glaze (1 serving/27g) 97 cals	5	0
Icing: vanilla, made with butter (1 serving/48g) 165 cals	9	0
Icing: vanilla, made with margarine (1 serving/48g) 194 cals	12	0

	RiskPoints ✗	LifePoints ✔
Jam tarts: (1 tart/40g) 154 cals	17	1
Lemon curd: (1 tbsp/20g) 58 cals	10	0
Lemon meringue pie: (1 serving/ 113g) 303 cals	24	5
Madeira cake: (1 serving/74g) 291 cals	48	2
Mince pies: (1 individual pie/ 50g) 218 cals	29	2
Pie crust: short-crust, baked (1 serving/23g) 121 cals	19	2
Pineapple upside-down cake: (1 serving/115g) 367 cals	34	7
Pound cake: made with butter (1 serving/53g) 229 cals	57	4
Puff pastry: baked (1oz/28g) 158 cals	27	2
Rice pudding: canned (1 can/ 5oz/142g) 231 cals	26	4
Sponge cake: (1 serving/38g) 110 cals	2	3
Suet pudding: (1 serving/115g) 383 cals	87	5
Treacle tart: (1 serving/115g) 427 cals	47	4
Trifle: (1 serving/115g) 184 cals	24	4

Dressings and Sauces

	RiskPoints ✗	LifePoints ✔
Barbecue sauce (½ cup/4 fl oz 125g) 94 cals	5	3
Bolognaise sauce (¾ cup/6 fl oz 200g) 278 cals	54	21

	RiskPoints ✗	LifePoints ✔
Cheese sauce: made with milk (½ cup/4 fl oz/140g) 154 cals	35	9
Hollandaise sauce: made with milk and butter (1 cup/8 fl oz/254g) 703 cals	313	9
Ketchup (1 tbsp/15g) 16 cals	2	0
Mayonnaise: made without dairy products (i.e. vegan) (1 tbsp/14g) 67 cals	16	0
Mayonnaise: made with soya bean oil (1 tbsp/13g) 99 cals	27	0
Mornay sauce: (½ cup/168g) 242 cals	64	15
Mustard: plain (1 tbsp/17g) 40 cals	6	2
Mustard: prepared with cream (1 tbsp/17g) 28 cals	9	0
Pickle: sweet (1 tbsp/15g) 20 cals	2	0
Salad dressing: blue and Roquefort cheese (1 tbsp/15g) 77 cals	20	0
Salad dressing: French (1 tbsp/14g) 88 cals	24	0
Salad dressing: French, low-fat (1 tbsp/16g) 22 cals	2	0
Salad dressing: Italian, low-fat (1 tbsp/15g) 16 cals	3	0
Salad dressing: Thousand Island (1 tbsp/15g) 59 cals	13	0
Salad dressing: Thousand Island, low-fat (1 tbsp/15g) 24 cals	4	0
Salad dressing: vinegar and oil (1 tbsp/15g) 70 cals	19	0
Sesame seed dressing: (1 tbsp/15g) 68 cals	17	0

	RiskPoints ✗	LifePoints ✔
Sweet and sour sauce: (½ cup/ 4 fl oz/156g) 147 cals	0	2
Tartar sauce: (1 tbsp/20g) 61 cals	12	0
Teriyaki sauce: (1 tbsp/18g) 15 cals	0	0
White sauce: made with milk (½ cup/4 fl oz/131g) 119 cals	23	7

Snacks and Sweets

	RiskPoints ✗	LifePoints ✔
Banana chips: (1oz/28g) 147 cals	61	1
Bread pudding: (½ cup/126g) 212 cals	21	7
Butterscotch or caramel topping: (2 tbsp/41g) 103 cals	0	0
Caramel cookie bar: (1 pkg/57g) 272 cals	33	3
Carob cookie: (1 bar/3oz/87g) 464 cals	71	17
Chips: see 'Potato chips' in the Vegetables and Vegetable Products group		
Chocolate pudding: made with whole milk (½ cup/142g) 158 cals	22	6
Chocolate: after dinner mints (2 pieces/8g) 29 cals	4	0
Chocolate: baking chocolate, unsweetened (1 square/1oz/28g) 148 cals	69	3
Chocolate: caramels in milk chocolate (1 pkg/55g) 261 cals	29	4
Chocolate: fudge (1 piece/17g) 65 cals	6	0

	RiskPoints ✗	LifePoints ✔
Chocolate: milk (1 bar/44g) 226 cals	60	4
Chocolate: milk chocolate coated peanuts (10 pieces/40g) 208 cals	43	5
Chocolate: milk chocolate coated raisins (10 pieces/10g) 39 cals	6	0
Chocolate: semi-sweet chocolate, made with butter (1oz/28g) 135 cals	37	1
Chocolate: semi-sweet chocolate, regular (1oz/28g) 135 cals	37	1
Chocolate: snack bar (1 bar/ 2.1oz/60g) 251 cals	35	4
Chocolate: sweet chocolate (1oz/ 28g) 143 cals	42	1
Chocolate: wafer bar (1 bar/ 1.6oz/46g) 235 cals	57	4
Crisps: barbecue flavoured (1oz/ 28g) 139 cals	22	4
Crisps: made from dried potatoes, lower fat (1oz/28g) 142 cals	18	3
Crisps: made from dried potatoes, regular (1oz/28g) 158 cals	27	2
Crisps: regular (1oz/28g) 152 cals	24	3
Crisps: sour cream and onion flavour (1oz/28g) 151 cals	24	5
Fish and chips: see 'Fish' in the Meat, Fish and Dairy group		
Fish fillet: see 'Fish' in the Meat, Fish and Dairy group		
Fish fingers: see 'Fish' in the Meat, Fish and Dairy group		
Fruit leather bar: (1 bar/23g) 81 cals	6	0

	RiskPoints ✗	LifePoints ✔
Ice cream: chocolate (1 serving/ 66g) 143 cals	40	4
Ice cream: strawberry (1 serving/ 66g) 127 cals	13	3
Ice cream: vanilla, regular (1 serving/66g) 133 cals	40	3
Ice cream: vanilla, rich (1 serving/74g) 178 cals	55	3
Ice cream: vanilla, soft-serve (1 serving/86g) 185 cals	48	5
Ice cream: yogurt, soft-serve (1 serving/72g) 114 cals	18	4
Ices: sorbet, made with water and fruit only (1 serving/96g) 75 cals	0	0
Jellies: (1 packet/14g) 38 cals	4	0
Jellybeans: (10 small/14g) 40 cals	5	0
Marmalade: orange (1 tbsp/20g) 49 cals	5	0
Marshmallows: (1 regular/7g) 23 cals	2	0
Molasses: blackstrap (1 tbsp/20g) 47 cals	0	5
Molasses: regular (1 tbsp/20g) 53 cals	2	1
Moussaka: see 'Lamb' in the Meat, Fish and Dairy group		
Muesli bar: (1 bar/24g) 115 cals	12	2
Nachos: with cheese (6–8 nachos/113g) 346 cals	58	14
Nachos: with cheese, beans, ground beef and peppers (6–8 nachos 255g) 569 cals	93	25
Pancakes: see 'Cooked Breakfast Foods' in the Cereals, Grains and Pasta group		

	RiskPoints ✗	LifePoints ✔
Peanut bar: (1 bar/45g) 235 cals	37	6
Peanut brittle: (1oz/28g) 128 cals	13	3
Pizza: *see* 'Breads' in the Cereals, Grains and Pasta group		
Popcorn: air-popped (1 cup/8g) 31 cals	0	1
Popcorn: caramel-coated (1 cup/ 35g) 152 cals	11	1
Popcorn: cheese flavour (1 cup/ 11g) 58 cals	9	1
Popcorn: oil-popped (1 cup/11g) 55 cals	7	1
Potato sticks: (1oz/28g) 148 cals	24	3
Pretzels: hard, salted (10 twists/ 60g) 229 cals	5	11
Sesame bar, brittle-type: (1oz/ 28g) 147 cals	23	7
Shepherd's pie: *see* 'Lamb' in the Meat, Fish and Dairy group		
Syrup: chocolate (2 tbsp/1fl oz 37g) 82 cals	1	0
Syrup: malt (1 tbsp/24g) 76 cals	9	2
Syrup: maple (1 tbsp/20g) 52 cals	4	0
Syrup: pancake (1 tbsp/20g) 57 cals	4	0
Taco salad: (1½ cups/198g) 279 cals	51	16
Taco salad with chilli con carne: (1½ cups/261g) 290 cals	45	22
Tapioca pudding: made with whole milk (½ cup/141g) 161 cals	19	5
Toffee: (1 piece/12g) 65 cals	18	0

	RiskPoints ✗	LifePoints ✔
Tortilla chips: nacho flavour (1oz/28g) 141 cals	18	2
Tortilla chips: plain (1oz/28g) 142 cals	18	2
Trail mix: (1oz/28g) 131 cals	20	5
Welsh rarebit: *see* 'Cheese' in the Meat, Fish and Dairy section		

Margarines, Oils and Spreads

	RiskPoints ✗	LifePoints ✔
For butter and butter oil (ghee) look under 'Dairy' in the Meat, Fish and Dairy group		
Almond oil: (1 tbsp/13.6g) 120 cals	34	0
Corn oil: salad or cooking (1 tbsp/13.6g) 120 cals	34	0
Hazelnut oil: (1 tbsp/13.6g) 120 cals	34	0
Margarine/butter: blend of 60 per cent corn oil margarine and 40 per cent butter (1 tsp/5g) 36 cals	10	0
Margarine: hard, made with hydrogenated oil (1 tsp/4g) 34 cals	9	0
Margarine: low-fat (approx 40 per cent made with hydrogenated soya bean oil (1 tsp/4g) 17 cals	4	0
Margarine: soft, made with hydrogenated or non-hydrogenated oil (1 tsp/4g) 34 cals	9	0
Olive oil: salad or cooking (1 tbsp/13.5g) 119 cals	33	0

	RiskPoints ✗	LifePoints ✔
Peanut oil: salad or cooking (1 tbsp/13g) 119 cals	33	0
Sesame oil: salad or cooking (1 tbsp/13g) 120 cals	34	0
Soya bean oil: salad or cooking (1 tbsp/13.6g) 120 cals	34	0
Sunflower oil: salad or cooking (1 tbsp/13.6g) 120 cals	34	0
Vegetable shortening: made with hydrogenated soya bean and palm oils (1 tbsp/12g) 113 cals	32	0
Walnut oil: (1 tbsp/13.6g) 120 cals	34	0
Wheat germ oil: (1 tbsp/13.6g) 120 cals	34	0

Herbs and Spices

	RiskPoints ✗	LifePoints ✔
Basil: fresh (5 leaves/2g) 1 cals	0	0
Basil: ground (1 tsp/1g) 4 cals	0	0
Bay leaf: crumbled (1 tsp/1g) 2 cals	0	0
Cardamon: ground (1 tsp/2g) 6 cals	0	0
Chilli powder: (1 tsp/2g) 8 cals	1	1
Cinnamom: ground (1 tsp/2g) 6 cals	0	1
Cloves: ground (1 tsp/2g) 7 cals	1	0
Coriander: fresh (¼ cup/4g) 1 cal	0	0
Cumin seed: (1 tsp/2g) 8 cals	1	1
Dill weed: fresh (5 sprigs/1g) 1 cal	0	0

	RiskPoints ✗	LifePoints ✔
Fennel seed: (1 tsp/2g) 7 cals	0	0
Ginger: ground (1 tsp/1g) 6 cals	0	0
Marjoram: dried (1 tsp/1g) 2 cals	0	0
Nutmeg: ground (1 tsp/2g) 12 cals	4	0
Oregano: ground (1 tsp/1g) 5 cals	0	0
Paprika: (1 tsp/2g) 6 cals	0	1
Parsley: dried (1 tsp/1g) 1 cal	0	0
Parsley: fresh (10 sprigs/10g) 4 cals	0	1
Pepper: black (1 tsp/2g) 5 cals	0	0
Poppy seed: (1 tsp/2g) 15 cals	3	1
Rosemary: dried (1 tsp/1g) 4 cals	0	0
Sage: ground (1 tsp/1g) 2 cals	0	0
Tarragon: ground (1 tsp/1g) 5 cals	0	0
Thyme: ground (1 tsp/1g) 4 cals	0	1
Turmeric: ground (1 tsp/2g) 8 cals	0	0

YOUR LIFEPOINTS DAILY PLANNER

DATE:

FOOD AND NOTES	Food Group	RiskPoints ✗	LifePoints ✔
TOTAL FOR THE DAY:			

REFERENCES

1 The Associated Press, 17 July 1994, *The Independent*, 24 March 1994.
2 Wooley, S.C. et al., *British Medical Journal* 1994; 309 n.6955 p.655(2).
3 National Academy of Science's figure, quoted by The Associated Press, 6 December 1994.
4 Gortmaker, S.L. et al., *N Engl J Med* 1993; 329:1008–12.
5 American Dietetic Association 1994 'How Are Americans Making Food Choices?'
6 Department of Health 1994 'Nutritional Aspects of Cardiovascular Disease'.
7 *The Women's Letter*, June 1990 v.3 n.6 p.1(2).
8 *Science News*, 1994 v.146 n.23 p.372(1).
9 *Consumer Reports*, June 1993.
10 The Associated Press, 2 August 1995.
11 *The Independent*, 1 August 1995.
12 *Tufts University Diet & Nutrition Letter*, 1995 v.13 n.1 p.1(2).
13 *The Independent*, 28 July 1995.
14 Lichtman, S.W. et al., *N Engl J Med* 1992; 327(27):1893–8.
15 *Merck Manual*, 16th edition, 1992.
16 *Consumer Reports*, June 1993.
17 Keys, A. et al., *J Chronic Dis* 1972; 25:329.
18 Classifications from Department of Health 1994 'Nutritional Aspects of Cardiovascular Disease'.
19 The Associated Press, 19 March 1994.
20 Rookus, M.A. et al., *Int J of Obes* 1988; n. 12, pp. 29–39.
21 Rookus, M.A. et al., *Int J Obes* 1988; n. 12, pp. 29–39.
22 Department of Health 1994 'Nutritional Aspects of Cardiovascular Disease'.
23 The Associated Press, 14 June 1994.
24 Abraham, S. et al., *Weight by height and age for adults 18–74 years*. National Center for Health Statistics 1979 *and* USDA Economics, Statistical and Cooperative Service, *Food consumption, prices and expenditures*, US GPO 1976.
25 E.G., inter alia, Wierzuchowski, M. et al., *J. Biol. Chem* 1925; 64: 697–707.
26 Pembry, M.S., *J. Physiol.* 1902; 27: 407–417.
27 Flatt, J.P., 'The biochemistry of energy expenditure' in: *Obesity Research II*, edited by G.A. Bray. London: Newman, 1978, pp.211–228.

28 Acheson, K.J. et al., *Metabolism* 1982; 31: 1234–40.

29 *The New York Times*, 24 March 1987.

30 Schutz, Y. et al., *Am J Clin Nutr* 1989; 50(2): 307–14.

31 *The New York Times*, 8 May 1990.

32 Beilin, L.J., *Clin. Exp. Hypertens.* [A] 1992; 14 (1–2) 213–21.

33 Collier, G. et al., *Diabetologia* 1984; 26: 50–54. Gulliford, M.C. et al., *Am. J. Clin. Nutr.* 1989; 50: 773–77. Gatti, E. et al., *Eur. J. Clin. Nutr.* 1991: 46: 161–66.

34 Forsgren, L., *Arch. Kemi* 1968; 30: 355–60. Watkins, J.B. et al., *Gastroenterol* 1982; 82: 911–2717. Jones, P.J.H. et al., *Am. J. Clin. Nutr.* 1985; 42: 769–77. Jones, P.J.H. et al., *Metabolism* 1992; 41: 396–401.

35 *Tufts University Diet & Nutrition Letter* 1995 v.13 n.3 p.4(3).

36 Otto, H. et al., *Diatetik bei Diabetes Mellitus.* Berne: Verlag Hans Huber, 1973 pp.41–50.

37 Yetiv, J., *Popular Nutritional Practices: A Scientific Appraisal*, Popular Medicine Press (US) 1986.

38 Wolever, T.M.S. et al., *Am J Clin Nutr* 1991; 54(5): 846–54.

39 Trout, D.L. et al., *Am J Clin Nutr* 1993; 58(6): 873–8.

40 Wolever, T.M.S. et al., *Am J Clin Nutr* 1991; 54(5): 846–54.

41 Trout, D.L. et al., *Am J Clin Nutr* 1993; 58(6): 873–8.

42 Jenkins, D.J. et al., *N Engl J Med* 1989; 321(14): 929–34.

43 Based on a lecture given to the Royal Society of Health.

44 Harman, D. *Proc Natl Acad Sci* 1991; 88: 5360–5363.

45 *Science* 1990; 250: 634–640.

46 Harman, D. *Proc Natl Acad Sci* 1991; 88: 5360–5363.

47 'Free radicals: from basic science to medicine', Birkhauser Verlag, Basel 1993.

48 Media statement, *Alliance for Aging Research*, 3 March 1994.

49 UPI, March 19, 1988

50 *Krause's Food Nutrition and Diet Therapy*, 8th edition, W.B. Saunders Company (US).

51 Kendall, A. et al., *Am J Clin Nutr* 1991; 53(5): 1124–9.

52 Barnard, N., *Food For Life*, Harmony Books 1993.

53 Himms-Hagen J., *Can Med Assoc J* 1979; 121: 1361.

54 Welle, S. et al., *Metabolism* 1980; 29(9): 806–9.

55 *The New York Times*, 22 May 1991.

56 Kendall, A. et al., *Am J Clin Nutr* 1991; 53(5): 1124–9.

57 Suter, P.M. et al., *New Engl J Med* 1992; 326: 983–87.

58 Willett, W.C., *Science* v.264, 22 April 1994.

INDEX